Thyroid For Dum***ies***

D0607793

Maximizing Your Thyroid Health

For more information about these steps, see Chapter 21:

- ✔ Ask your doctor to screen you for thyroid disease at appropriate intervals; I recommend being screened every five years beginning at age 35.
- ✔ Check your thyroid function during times of major body changes, such as pregnancy.
- ✔ Make sure that you get enough iodine in your diet, especially if you are a vegetarian.
- ✔ If you've been taking thyroid hormone replacement for several years to treat *hypothyroidism* (low thyroid function), ask your doctor if you can try stopping treatment to see if your thyroid can function without it.
- ✔ If you still experience symptoms of hypothyroidism while taking hormone replacement pills, ask your doctor if you can try taking a pill that contains both types of thyroid hormone (T4 and T3).
- ✔ Be aware of medications that can interact with thyroid hormones. (For a complete discussion of drug interactions, see Chapter 10.)
- ✔ Protect your thyroid from radiation. If your neck has been exposed to radiation in the past, be sure that your doctor knows that.
- ✔ Be aware of new discoveries in thyroid health and treatment. Appendix B features many Web sites that can help you do this.

Signs and Symptoms of Low Thyroid Function

Someone with *hypothyroidism* — a low functioning thyroid — often experiences some of the following signs and symptoms. (Keep in mind that these symptoms alone can't diagnose thyroid disease, and thyroid disease may be present even if you don't experience all these symptoms. See Chapter 5 for detailed information about hypothyroidism.)

- ✔ Slow pulse
- ✔ Enlarged thyroid (unless it has been removed during prior thyroid treatment)
- ✔ Dry, cool skin that is puffy, pale, and yellowish
- ✔ Brittle nails and dry, brittle hair that falls out excessively
- ✔ Swelling, especially of the legs
- ✔ Hoarseness, slow speech, and a thickened tongue
- ✔ Slow reflexes
- ✔ Intolerance to cold
- ✔ Tiredness and a need to sleep excessively
- ✔ Constipation
- ✔ Increased menstrual flow

Signs and Symptoms of Excessive Thyroid Function

Someone with *hyperthyroidism* — excessive thyroid function — may experience some or all of the following symptoms. (The same caution about symptoms of hypothyroidism applies here; these symptoms alone don't confirm a diagnosis. Only lab tests ordered by your doctor can do that. See Chapter 6 for more information about hyperthyroidism.)

- Higher body temperature and intolerance to heat
- Weight loss
- Weakness
- Enlarged thyroid
- Warm, moist skin
- Rapid pulse
- Tremors of the fingers and tongue
- Increased reflexes
- Nervousness
- Difficulty sleeping
- Rapid mood changes
- Decreased menstrual flow
- More frequent bowel movements
- Changes to the eyes that make it appear as if you're staring

Medications to Watch Out For

Certain drugs can interact with your thyroid hormone to negatively affect your thyroid function. Chapter 10 goes into detail about this subject, but following are just a few commonly used medications that can impact your thyroid:

- Amiodarone
- Aspirin (more than 3,000 milligrams daily)
- Estrogen
- Iron tablets
- Iodine
- Lithium
- Propranolol
- Steroids

For Dummies: Bestselling Book Series for Beginners

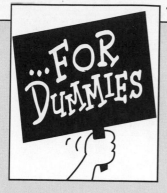

™

References for the Rest of Us!®

BESTSELLING BOOK SERIES

Do you find that traditional reference books are overloaded with technical details and advice you'll never use? Do you postpone important life decisions because you just don't want to deal with them? Then our *For Dummies*® business and general reference book series is for you.

For Dummies business and general reference books are written for those frustrated and hard-working souls who know they aren't dumb, but find that the myriad of personal and business issues and the accompanying horror stories make them feel helpless. *For Dummies* books use a lighthearted approach, a down-to-earth style, and even cartoons and humorous icons to dispel fears and build confidence. Lighthearted but not lightweight, these books are perfect survival guides to solve your everyday personal and business problems.

"More than a publishing phenomenon, 'Dummies' is a sign of the times."

— The New York Times

"A world of detailed and authoritative information is packed into them…"

— U.S. News and World Report

"…you won't go wrong buying them."

— Walter Mossberg, Wall Street Journal, on For Dummies books

Already, millions of satisfied readers agree. They have made For Dummies the #1 introductory level computer book series and a best-selling business book series. They have written asking for more. So, if you're looking for the best and easiest way to learn about business and other general reference topics, look to For Dummies to give you a helping hand.

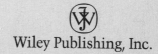

Wiley Publishing, Inc.

5/09

Thyroid
FOR
DUMMIES®

by Alan L. Rubin, M.D.

Wiley Publishing, Inc.

Thyroid For Dummies®

Published by
Wiley Publishing, Inc.
909 Third Avenue
New York, NY 10022
www.wiley.com

Copyright © 2001 by Wiley Publishing, Inc., Indianapolis, Indiana

About the Author

Alan L. Rubin, M.D., is one of the nation's foremost experts on the thyroid gland in health and disease. He is a member of the Endocrine Society and has been in private practice specializing in thyroid disease and diabetes for over 28 years. Dr. Rubin was Assistant Clinical Professor of Medicine at UC Medical Center in San Francisco for 20 years. He has spoken about the thyroid to professional medical audiences and non-medical audiences around the world. He is a consultant to many pharmaceutical companies and companies that make thyroid products.

Dr. Rubin has written extensively on the thyroid gland as well as diabetes mellitus. As a result, he has been on numerous radio and television programs, talking about the cause, the prevention, and the treatment of conditions of the thyroid. He is also the best-selling author of *Diabetes For Dummies* and *Diabetes Cookbook For Dummies.*

Dedication

This book is dedicated to my wife, Enid, who was there for every page. She smilingly let me do my work, sometimes into the wee hours of the morning, and missed many an opportunity to go out to dinner or a movie so that I could produce this book for you. If you have a fraction of the support in your life that she has given me, you are a lucky person, indeed.

Author's Acknowledgments

The great publisher and midwife, Kathy Nebenhaus, deserves enormous appreciation for helping me to deliver yet another bright-eyed baby. Her optimism and her enthusiasm actually made this book possible. Her assistant, Natasha Graf, played a huge role in ironing out the inevitable problems that arise when book-publishing and medicine meet.

My editor, Joan Friedman, did a magnificent job turning my sometimes-incomprehensible prose into words that you can understand. She also conducted a whole orchestra of other editors who contributed to the book, including Robert Annis, Christy Beck, Mary Fales, Alison Jefferson, and Greg Pearson.

My thanks to Dr. Catherine Bain for the technical editing of the book.

Librarians Mary Ann Zaremska and Nancy Phelps at St. Francis Memorial Hospital were tremendously helpful in providing the articles and books upon which the information in this book is based.

My teachers are too numerous to mention, but one person deserves special attention. Dr. Francis Greenspan at the University of California Medical Center gave me the sound foundation in thyroid function and disease upon which this book is based.

Finally, there are my patients over the last 28 years, the people whose trials and tribulations caused me to seek the knowledge that you will find in this book.

This book is written on the shoulders of thousands of men and women who made the discoveries, tried the medications, and held the committee meetings. Their accomplishments cannot possibly be given adequate acclaim. We owe them big time.

Publisher's Acknowledgments

We're proud of this book; please send us your comments through our online registration form located at www.dummies.com/register.

Some of the people who helped bring this book to market include the following:

Acquisitions, Editorial, and Media Development

Senior Project Editor: Joan Friedman

Acquisitions Editors: Stacy Collins, Tracy Boggier

Copy Editors: Robert Annis, Mary Fales, Greg Pearson

Technical Editor: Catherine Bain, M.D.

Editorial Manager: Christine Meloy Beck

Editorial Assistant: Jennifer Young

Cover Photo: © Custom Medical Stock Photo

Production

Project Coordinator: Jennifer Bingham

Layout and Graphics: Jackie Nicholas, Jacque Schneider, Jeremey Unger

Special Art: Kathryn Born, Medical Illustrator

Proofreaders: Betty Kish, Marianne Santy

Indexer: Liz Cunningham

Special Help
Alison Jefferson

Publishing and Editorial for Consumer Dummies
Diane Graves Steele, Vice President and Publisher, Consumer Dummies
Joyce Pepple, Acquisitions Director, Consumer Dummies
Kristin A. Cocks, Product Development Director, Consumer Dummies
Michael Spring, Vice President and Publisher, Travel
Brice Gosnell, Publishing Director, Travel
Suzanne Jannetta, Editorial Director, Travel

Publishing for Technology Dummies
Andy Cummings, Acquisitions Director

Composition Services
Gerry Fahey, Executive Director of Production Services
Debbie Stailey, Director of Composition Services

Contents at a Glance

Cartoons at a Glance

By Rich Tennant

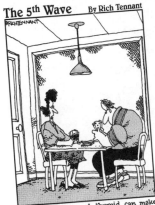

"Look—an abnormal thyroid can make you irritable, nervous, and weak in the upper arms. But you can't blame it for the rotten game of gin you're playing."

page 263

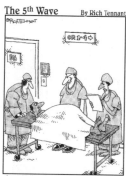

"Included with today's surgery, we're offering a manicure, pedicure, haircut, and ear wax flush for just $49.95."

page 239

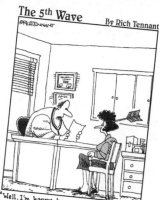

"Well, I'm happy to run some tests, but to be honest, I think it's all in your head."

page 7

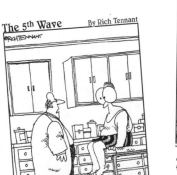

"Well, Mr. Humphrey—it appears your thyroid isn't the only thing that's become enlarged."

page 167

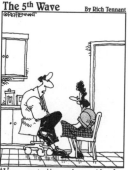

"Yes, perspiration and a rapid pulse could indicate hyperthyroidism. But the fact that these symptoms occur only when the pool boy is working in your backyard does raise some questions."

page 47

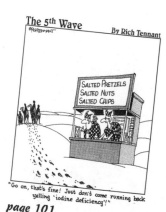

"Go on, that's fine! Just don't come running back yelling 'iodine deficiency'!"

page 101

Cartoon Information:
Fax: 978-546-7747
E-Mail: richtennant@the5thwave.com
World Wide Web: www.the5thwave.com

Table of Contents

Introduction

*A*s I entered the psychiatric medical unit at Bellevue Hospital the first day of my internship in 1966, I noticed a loud woman with penetrating eyes. I looked closely at her and saw that her neck was very enlarged. Since I was the new doctor on the unit, I picked up her chart and discovered that she had a case of Graves' disease, a form of excessive thyroid production. For the next few months, I became intimately involved with her problems. She taught me a great deal about thyroid disease and probably represents the explanation for my lifelong interest in this subject. I have taken care of many such patients over the years (though never again in a psychiatric unit), but she stands out in my memory like a first love.

For hundreds of years, people have understood that a connection exists between a strange-looking growth in the neck and certain diseases. Until about 60 years ago, confusion reigned because people with similar growths in their necks often had opposite conditions. One group would show excessive excitement, nervousness, and shakiness, while the other would show depression, sleepiness, and general loss of interest. What the two groups had in common was that they consisted mostly of women.

Around 60 years ago, it became possible to measure the chemicals that were coming from those growths (which were enlarged thyroid glands), and suddenly the whole picture began to make sense. Since then, a vast amount has been learned about the thyroid, the chemicals (hormones) made in that gland, and the purpose of those hormones.

In this book you will benefit from the hard work of doctors and other scientists over the last few hundred years. You will find that with very rare exceptions, thyroid diseases, including thyroid cancer, are some of the most easily treated of all disorders. (This is why many thyroid specialists say, "If I have to have a cancer, let it be a thyroid cancer.")

After you read this book, I hope you will be a lot less confused than the poor thyroid itself, which doesn't know where it is. I once heard the left side of a thyroid say to the right, "We must be in Capistrano. Here comes another swallow."

If you've read either of my previous books, *Diabetes For Dummies* or *Diabetes Cookbook For Dummies,* you know that I use humor to get my ideas across, a technique that characterizes the *For Dummies* series. I want to emphasize that I'm not trying to trivialize anyone's suffering by being comic about it. The work of Norman Cousins and others has shown that humor has healing properties. A positive attitude is far more conducive to a positive outcome than is a negative attitude.

About This Book

I don't expect you to read this book from cover to cover. Since the first few chapters are a general introduction to the thyroid, you may want to start in Part I, but if you prefer to go right to information about the thyroid condition that affects you, by all means do so. If you run across any terms that you don't understand, look for them in the glossary of terms in Appendix A.

I've written this book as a sort of medical biography of the Dummy family — Tami Dummy, Stacy Dummy, Linda Dummy, Ken Dummy, and other members of the clan whom you'll meet during your reading. These folks illustrate the fact that thyroid disease often runs in families. (There are exceptions to this fact, which I explain.) You meet members of the Dummy family, as well as some other fine fictional folks, at the beginning of each chapter that describes a thyroid disease, so that you have a good picture of the condition covered in that chapter.

Conventions Used in This Book

As much as I would love to use all nonscientific terms in this book, if I did so, you and your doctor would be speaking two different languages. Therefore, I do use scientific terms, but I explain them in everyday English the first time you run across them. Plus, those difficult terms are defined in the glossary at the back of the book.

Three scientific terms come up over and over again in this book: *thyroxine, triiodothyronine,* and *thyroid-stimulating hormone* (also known as *thyrotropin*). These terms are explained in detail in Chapter 3. For these three words, I often use abbreviations: Thyroxine is T4, triiodothyronine is T3, and thyroid-stimulating hormone is TSH.

What You Don't Have to Read

Throughout the book, you find shaded boxes of text called *sidebars*. These contain material that is interesting but not essential to your understanding. If you don't care to go so deeply into a subject, skip the sidebars; you can still understand everything else.

Assumptions

I make the assumption in this book that you or someone you care about has a thyroid condition that has not been treated or perhaps is not being treated to your satisfaction. If this assumption doesn't apply to you, perhaps you suspect that you have a thyroid condition and want to determine whether you should see a doctor, or you can't get your doctor to run the necessary tests to determine whether a thyroid problem exists. Regardless of your individual situation, this book has valuable information for you.

I try to make no assumptions about what you know related to the thyroid. I don't introduce any new terms without explaining what they are. If you already know a lot about the thyroid and its functions, you can still find new information that adds to your knowledge.

How This Book Is Organized

The book is divided into six parts to help you find out all you want to know about the thyroid gland.

Part 1: Understanding the Thyroid

So much (right and wrong) has been written about the way the thyroid affects your mood that I thought I would clear up this subject at the very beginning of the book. After you understand how the thyroid affects your emotions, you find out just what the thyroid is and what it does. Finally, in this part you learn about the medical tests that help us determine if something is wrong with your thyroid.

Part II: What's Wrong with My Thyroid?

This part explains each of the conditions that affect the thyroid and how they affect you. By the time you finish with this part of the book, I may be able to retire, because you will know just about everything I know about thyroid disease, how to identify it, and how to treat it.

Part III: Managing Your Thyroid

Here you discover how medications you take can influence your thyroid function. I also explain thyroid infections, along with the worldwide problem of iodine deficiency. Finally, I show you why thyroid surgery is rarely done and what new treatments are coming along.

Part IV: Special Considerations in Thyroid Health

Three groups of people deserve special consideration in this book: pregnant women, children, and the elderly. Thyroid conditions take unusual directions in these groups, so the chapters in this part address their unique difficulties. The final chapter here offers suggestions for ways to improve your thyroid health — and your health in general — through diet, exercise, and lifestyle choices.

Part V: The Part of Tens

Misinformation about the thyroid is rampant. In this part, I clear up some of that misinformation (though not all, because it accumulates faster than I can address it). I also show you how you can maximize your thyroid health.

Part VI: Appendixes

In Appendix A, you find a glossary of medical terms that relate to the thyroid; you may want to bookmark it so you can go back and forth with ease as you read other chapters. In Appendix B, I direct you to the best-of-the-best Web sites where you can get dependable facts to fill in any blank spots that remain after you've read this book.

Icons Used in This Book

Books in the *For Dummies* series feature icons in the margins, which direct you toward information that may be of particular interest or importance. Here's an explanation of what each icon in this book signifies:

When you see this icon, it means the information is essential. You want to be sure you understand it.

This icon points out important information that can save you time and energy.

You find this icon next to paragraphs in which I tell you about the Dummy family or other folks with specific thyroid conditions.

This icon alerts you to situations in which you may need to dial up your doctor for some help.

This icon warns against potential problems you could encounter, such as the side effects of mixing medications.

I define medical terms where you see this icon.

Where to Go from Here

Where you go from here depends upon your needs. If you want to understand how the thyroid works, head to Part I. If you or someone you know has a thyroid condition, you may want to pay particular attention to Part II. For help in maintaining good thyroid health, turn to Part III. If you are pregnant or have a child or parent with a thyroid disorder, Part IV is your next stop. In any case, as my mother used to say when she gave me a present, use this book in good health.

If you've had an unusual or even a humorous thyroid experience you'd like to share, by all means, let me know about it by e-mailing me at thyroid@drrubin.com. Who knows, I may share it with the world in a future edition of this book.

Part I

Understanding the Thyroid

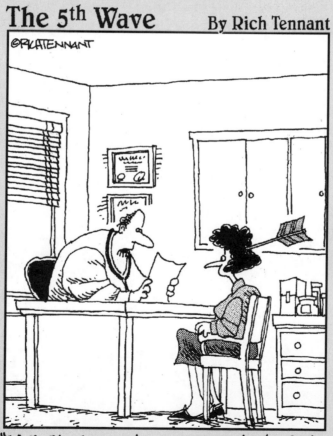

The 5th Wave   By Rich Tennant

"Well, I'm happy to run some tests, but to be honest, I think it's all in your head."

In this part . . .

What, exactly, is the thyroid gland, and what does it do? In this part, you discover how important this little gland in your neck really is, what function it plays in your body, and how to determine if it is functioning properly. I show you that your thyroid affects your mind as well as your body in critical ways.

Chapter 1

The Big Role of a Little Gland

- -

In This Chapter

▶ Crunching numbers: The incidence of thyroid disease

▶ Recognizing signs, symptoms, and risk factors

▶ Appreciating your thyroid's hard work

▶ Giving a sick thyroid some TLC

▶ Pinpointing times of life that pose special risks

- -

The thyroid is a little like Rodney Dangerfield: It doesn't get the respect it deserves. Anyone who watches those primetime TV news shows knows about the importance of other body parts — the heart and lungs sure get a lot of press time. But unless you come face-to-face with a thyroid problem, chances are that you don't hear much about what this little gland does and how important it is to your good health.

The fact that you're reading these words tells me that you've encountered a thyroid problem personally. (I suppose it's possible that you just picked this book up off the shelf out of curiosity — or because you belong to the Dr. Rubin Fan Club — but I'm betting that a thyroid problem is the more likely impetus.) Maybe you've recently been diagnosed with a thyroid condition. Or maybe your husband, wife, mother, or friend is being treated for a thyroid problem. You've probably found out at least a little about this mysterious gland. Now you're looking for answers to the questions that keep popping up in your mind:

- What causes this condition?

- What types of symptoms are related to this problem?

- How is this condition treated?

- What are the consequences of leaving it untreated?

- Does treatment end the problem forever?

- What can I (or my husband, wife, mother, or friend) do to help get back to optimal health?

I can't promise that this book will give you every possible answer to your questions. After all, doctors and researchers are constantly discovering new things about the thyroid — the information here is only as complete as our current knowledge. But if you're looking for concrete information about how the thyroid functions, what makes it malfunction, and what to do when a problem occurs, you're holding the right book.

Discovering the Extent of the Problem

Thyroid disease may be one of the most common diseases in the world. Research has indicated that thyroid disease affects more than 200 million people worldwide. Table 1-1 shows the approximate incidence, in 2001, of various types of thyroid disease in the United States, which has a population of more than 275 million. (*Incidence* means the number of new cases found in a year.)

Table 1-1	Incidence of Thyroid Disorders in the U.S.
Hypothyroidism (low thyroid function)	1.75 million
Hyperthyroidism (excessive thyroid function)	275,000
Goiter (enlarged thyroid)	22 million
Cancer	15,000
Death due to thyroid cancer	2,000

The incidence of thyroid disease becomes even higher when careful autopsies are done on people who did not die of a thyroid condition. As many as 60 percent of these people are found to have growths on the thyroid, and 17 percent have small areas of cancer that were not detected during life.

These numbers are statistics, but thyroid disease affects individuals. It may help to realize that many people in the public eye have gone on to great accomplishments after being treated successfully for thyroid conditions. Some of the people you may recognize include the following:

- Model Kim Alexis had hypothyroidism.
- Author Isaac Asimov had thyroid cancer.
- Golfers Pat Bradley and Ben Crenshaw both had hyperthyroidism.
- Former President George Bush, former first lady Barbara Bush, and even their dog Millie had hyperthyroidism.

✔ Runner Gail Devers had hyperthyroidism, while runner Carl Lewis had hypothyroidism.

✔ Former second lady Tipper Gore was treated for a thyroid growth, as was singer Rod Stewart.

I particularly enjoy the story of Isaac Asimov. He had thyroid cancer at age 52, and he died of unrelated causes at age 72. After his cancer surgery, he wrote about how he had paid $1,500 for the surgery and then wrote an article about the experience for which he received $2,000. Asimov said that he had the last laugh on the medical profession and was glad that he did not finish medical school.

This list is far from exhaustive, but it should help drive home the point that, if diagnosed and treated, thyroid conditions don't need to put a damper on your lifestyle.

Identifying an Unhappy Thyroid

Let's tackle some basics: Where is the thyroid, and how do you know when it needs some tender loving care? Chapter 3 gives you a detailed explanation of how to locate your thyroid, but for now, suffice it to say that it's just below your Adam's apple, at the front of your neck. If your thyroid becomes visible in your neck, if that area of your neck is tender, or if you have some trouble swallowing or breathing, you should consider visiting your doctor so that he or she can examine your thyroid. Any change in the size or shape of your thyroid can indicate that it's not functioning correctly or that you have growths on your thyroid called *nodules,* which should be tested to rule out cancer (see Chapter 7). Soreness or tenderness in the area of your thyroid may indicate that you have an infection or inflammation, which I discuss in Chapter 11.

In addition to changes in the size and shape of the gland, some very common problems occur when your thyroid malfunctions. If your thyroid function is low (you have *hypothyroidism*), you feel cold, tired, and maybe even a little depressed. I know that description doesn't sound very specific — those symptoms could indicate any number of other physical problems. But low thyroid function is so prevalent that it's worth asking your doctor to check it out if you experience such symptoms, especially if you are over the age of 35. Chapter 5 gives you the specifics about the causes and symptoms of hypothyroidism.

When your thyroid function is too high (you have *hyperthyroidism*), you feel hyper and warm, and your heart races. You may have trouble sitting still, and your emotions may change very rapidly for no clear reason. These symptoms are a little more specific than those for low thyroid function, but again, they could easily result from some cause not related to your thyroid. The best way to determine whether a thyroid problem exists is to ask your doctor to check your thyroid function. Chapter 6 offers a detailed look at hyperthyroidism.

Recognizing Who's at Risk

A few key facts help doctors determine whether thyroid disease is a strong probability for a given patient:

- ✔ Women are affected by thyroid problems much more frequently than men.
- ✔ Thyroid conditions tend to run in families.
- ✔ Thyroid problems often arise after the age of 30.

This doesn't mean that a 20-year-old man with no family history of thyroid problems can't develop a thyroid condition. It simply means that a 35-year-old woman whose mother was diagnosed with low thyroid function 20 years ago is at greater risk of having a thyroid problem than the young man is. With this in mind, the young woman should be sure to tell her doctor about her family history. And she should definitely be tested periodically to make sure her thyroid function is normal.

About half (perhaps even more) of all the people with thyroid disorders are undiagnosed. The American Thyroid Association and other experts recommend that thyroid testing begin at age 35 and continue every 5 years thereafter. Women with family histories of thyroid disease may benefit from even more frequent testing.

Realizing the Importance of a Healthy Thyroid

Your thyroid gland influences almost every cell and organ in your body because its general function is to control your metabolism. If your thyroid is functioning correctly, your metabolism should be normal. If your thyroid is working too hard, your metabolism is too high, and the result can be anything from an increased body temperature to an elevated heart rate. When your thyroid function drops below normal, so does your metabolism — you may gain weight, feel tired, and experience digestive problems.

Chapter 3 details how your thyroid affects various parts of your body, including your muscles, heart, lungs, stomach, intestines, skin, hair, nails, brain, bones, and sexual organs. (That's quite a list!)

As if that weren't enough, the thyroid also affects your mental health. People with low functioning thyroids often experience depression, while those with thyroids that work too hard can be jittery, irritable, and unable to concentrate. The mental and emotional consequences of a thyroid problem are so important, and so often misunderstood, that I've devoted all of Chapter 2 to exploring and explaining them. If I accomplish just one thing with this book, I hope I can raise your awareness of this important aspect of thyroid disease that can have such devastating effects if left undiagnosed and untreated.

Treating What Ails You

Depending on the specific thyroid problem, treatment options can range from taking a daily pill to having surgery to remove part or all of the thyroid. I discuss the details of treatment options, and I offer my opinions about which options are generally best, throughout Part I of this book. But keep in mind that no matter what you read here (or anywhere else), you should always discuss your specific situation with your doctor. This book can help you have a more productive conversation with your doctor by explaining the pros and cons of each type of treatment and by suggesting questions to ask your doctor if a treatment doesn't seem to be working for you. It cannot, however, act as a substitute for your doctor, because I don't know the ins and outs of your particular case.

In general, if you experience hypothyroidism (low thyroid function), your doctor will prescribe a daily pill to replace the thyroid hormone that your body is lacking. Many people take this type of pill for the rest of their lives, but some people are able to stop taking it after a few years if lab tests prove that the condition has righted itself. See Chapter 5 for a detailed discussion of treating hypothyroidism.

Three types of treatment options exist for someone with hyperthyroidism (an overactive thyroid). A patient with this condition may be placed on antithyroid drugs, may be given a dose of radioactive iodine in a pill in order to destroy part of the thyroid tissue, or may undergo surgery to remove some or all of the thyroid gland. In the United States, most doctors recommend the radioactive iodine treatment for this condition, but I have seen antithyroid drugs work very well for many patients. Surgery generally is performed only when a patient can't have one of the other two treatments. Chapter 6 goes into the specifics about each treatment and explains why your doctor may suggest one treatment over the others, depending on your specific situation.

For patients with thyroid cancer, surgery is often required. Radioactive iodine may also be used to destroy any thyroid tissue that remains after the surgery. Chapter 8 discusses the treatment of various types of thyroid cancer.

Someone whose thyroid has *nodules* (bumps) may need surgery, may not need treatment at all, or may need a type of treatment that falls between those extremes, such as thyroid hormone replacement or radioactive iodine. See Chapters 7 and 9 for all the details about how your doctor may deal with thyroid bumps and lumps.

The Consequences of Delaying Treatment

Earlier in the chapter, I mention that at least half of all people with thyroid conditions are undiagnosed. Many people die of other causes without ever discovering their thyroid problem. This statistic may lead you to wonder whether the diagnosis and treatment of thyroid problems is really necessary.

In some situations, a thyroid condition may be so benign that you don't even notice it. For example, many people with thyroid nodules never have any other problems except for a little bump on the neck. In those cases, treatment may be unnecessary.

But for many other people, thyroid conditions are much more serious, having a significant impact on overall health and quality of life. The section "Realizing the Importance of a Healthy Thyroid," earlier in this chapter, should give you a sense of what some consequences of delaying treatment may be. If you have a low functioning thyroid that is left untreated, you could become so fatigued and depressed that you'd have trouble just doing your daily activities. With an overactive thyroid, you could experience heart trouble and extreme nervousness. A cancerous thyroid could be life-threatening if untreated, depending on the type of cancer. And a thyroid with many nodules could become so enlarged or misshapen that it impacts your ability to swallow or breathe.

Unless your symptoms are already extreme, only lab tests can determine whether treatment for your thyroid condition is necessary. Given how important this little gland is to your health, both physical and mental, I can't imagine *not* asking your doctor to determine whether treatment is required.

Giving Your Thyroid a Hand: Healthy Lifestyle Choices

So you or a loved one has been diagnosed with a thyroid problem — what next? You start taking a prescription, or you undergo another type of treatment, and you wonder what else you should be doing to help yourself along toward better health. Is there something you did wrong that led to this problem in the first place? Is there some change you can make in your lifestyle that will lead to a cure?

I wish I could just tell you that if you ate more lima beans and got eight hours of sleep each night, your thyroid would return to perfect health. I could stop writing right now if that were the case. Unfortunately, the line between lifestyle choices and thyroid health isn't quite so straight. Your lifestyle definitely plays a role in your thyroid health, but lifestyle does not seem to cause thyroid conditions in the first place. If you are diagnosed with a hyperactive thyroid, for example, you most likely have the condition because you inherited a certain gene (or group of genes), as I discuss in Chapter 14. But if your life is full of stress, if you sleep only five hours a night, and if you drink lots of caffeine to get through the day, you definitely aren't doing your thyroid any favors. You may be aggravating the symptoms of your thyroid condition through your lifestyle choices; if you make some positive changes to your eating, sleeping, and exercise habits, your thyroid will definitely benefit.

In Chapter 19, I suggest ways that you can take a proactive role in upgrading your thyroid health by improving your diet, reducing your stress, exercising on a regular basis, and keeping a close eye on other aspects of your lifestyle.

Paying Special Attention: Pregnant Women, Children, and the Elderly

I believe that everyone should be tested periodically, especially after age 30, to ensure that their thyroids are working as they should. But certain groups of people need to pay special attention to their thyroid function. Pregnant women, children, and the elderly have even more at stake than other folks when it comes to monitoring thyroid function. For this reason, I've devoted Part IV of this book to these three groups.

Pregnancy can have a big impact on a woman's thyroid, whether she had a thyroid condition prior to the pregnancy or not. If she does have a known thyroid condition, her doctor will monitor it closely during pregnancy because her treatment may need to be altered. But if she doesn't have a thyroid condition, she and her doctor should watch carefully for signs and symptoms of thyroid problems, which can be triggered by the physiological changes she's experiencing.

Not only is a healthy thyroid crucial for the mother during pregnancy, but it's essential for the development of the fetus as well. For details about what to watch for during pregnancy, and the types of problems a thyroid condition can create for mother and child, see Chapter 16.

Chapter 17 discusses the importance of thyroid screening after the baby is born. Screening is mandatory by law because a healthy thyroid is necessary for proper mental and physical development. If you're a parent of an infant or young child, be sure to take a look at Chapter 17 so you understand what the screening is for, what risks are involved for children of parents with thyroid disease, and how those risks can be reduced.

The third group that should pay special attention to thyroid health is the elderly (for purposes of this discussion, people age 65 and over). The reason they are at such risk for thyroid disease is because the symptoms of a thyroid condition so often mirror symptoms of other ailments. If an elderly person is known to have a heart or blood pressure problem, a doctor may overlook a possible diagnosis of thyroid disease and attribute its symptoms to another condition. To confuse the issue even more, elderly people often experience symptoms that are *opposite* of what we expect to see with a certain thyroid condition. For example, an elderly person with a low functioning thyroid may actually lose weight (instead of gaining weight, which would be expected), because he or she is depressed and loses interest in food.

My goal is to help you preserve and defend your thyroid by knowing what to look for no matter what stage of life you're in. The more you know about the signs and symptoms of thyroid disease, the earlier you'll be able to alert your doctor that thyroid function tests may be a good idea.

Staying Informed

Doctors don't know everything. We do, however, tend to have an insatiable curiosity that drives us to always seek more information about the conditions we encounter. For this reason, new discoveries and treatment breakthroughs are popping up all the time. By the time this book is printed, hundreds of studies will have been conducted that suggest or prove something new about thyroid diseases and their treatment.

I can't update this book every time I discover something new, but you can still stay on top of the latest discoveries thanks to the speed of the Internet. In Appendix B, I direct you to electronic resources that you can use to stay up-to-date on thyroid health. If you use only one of these resources, I hope that it's my own Web page, www.drrubin.com, which can link you to all the other sites I recommend.

Chapter 2

The Thyroid and Your Mental Health

*T*he term *myxedema madness* may not be familiar to you, but it was popular when it was introduced in 1949 and for many years thereafter. *Myxedema* refers to low thyroid function, or hypothyroidism. The term *myxedema madness* resulted in the unfortunate association that all people with low thyroid function were somehow mad. My goal in this chapter is to clear up this misconception.

There's no question that the abnormal production of thyroid hormones, which I explain in Chapter 3, causes changes in the mood of a patient, which are sometimes severe. But only the rare patient has mood changes so severe that hospitalization is required. Most patients respond very well to treatment of an over- or underactive thyroid, and they live psychologically and physically normal lives.

In this chapter, I share what doctors currently understand about how changes in the production of thyroid hormones (both over- and underproduction) affect your personality. You discover how often personality or mood disorders are associated with thyroid abnormalities and why thyroid hormones play a role in the treatment of depression, even when no thyroid problem exists.

Because the emphasis in this chapter is on the psychology of thyroid abnormalities, I don't discuss physical signs and symptoms here; those discussions occur later in the book, especially in Chapters 5 and 6.

The Underactive Thyroid and Your Mood

Sarah Dummy is a 44-year-old woman who has not been herself for several months. Her husband, Milton, has noticed that she is much less talkative than before. She often forgets to pick up the food that they need at the supermarket or to stop at the dry cleaner's to pick up clothes she dropped off.

Milton has been wanting to discuss a vacation with Sarah, but she doesn't seem to care. Sarah is usually the one responsible for making plans with their friends, but she has not made any for months. Everything she does seems to take more time than it used to, like preparing dinner or getting ready to go to bed. When she finally gets in bed, she is not particularly interested in having sex anymore. The worst thing is that Sarah, usually a happy person, seems sad a lot of the time.

Worried about all these changes, Milton encourages Sarah to see Dr. Rubin, who examines her and sends her for some lab tests. On a return visit a few days later, Dr. Rubin tells them that Sarah has *hypothyroidism*. That is, her thyroid gland is not making enough thyroid hormone. He gives her a prescription for replacement thyroid hormone, and about a month later Sarah is well on her way to becoming her old self. Milton is happy because he has clean underwear again.

Sarah is an excellent example of the changes in personality that occur when the body is not producing enough thyroid hormone. Depending upon the level of the deficiency, the changes can be more or less severe. They include the following:

- Decreased talking
- Memory loss
- General loss of interest
- Withdrawal from society
- A general slowing of movement
- Depression, generally mild but sometimes severe
- Loss of interest in sex
- In severe cases, a kind of ironic sense of humor

No one or group of these mental changes means that you definitely have low thyroid function, but they certainly suggest that you need to be tested to find out.

If lack of thyroid hormone is determined to be the cause of these symptoms, then the right dose of hormone replacement should reverse them. If it does not, then you and your doctor need to look elsewhere for the cause. See Chapter 5 for a thorough discussion of hypothyroidism.

Overactivity of the Thyroid and Your Mind

Sarah Dummy's sister, Margaret, who is five years younger, began showing some big personality changes a few years ago. Previously a fairly even-tempered person, she now becomes easily excited and loses her temper after fairly mild provocation. Her small children never know when their mother is going to yell at them. She sometimes has a crying spell but, if asked, cannot give a reason why.

At other times, Margaret is extremely happy, but she can't explain the reason for that either. When she tries to do a task, she often loses interest rapidly and gets distracted. She cannot sit still for very long and seems to be always moving. Her memory of recent events is poor.

Margaret and her husband, Fred, go to see Dr. Rubin about her condition after a few months of absolute chaos in their home. During an examination, Dr. Rubin discovers a number of physical findings, including a rapid pulse, a large thyroid gland, and a fine tremor of Margaret's fingers. He confirms his findings with lab tests (see Chapter 4). Two days later, he tells the concerned pair that Margaret is suffering from *hyperthyroidism* — her body is producing too much thyroid hormone. He begins treatment with medication, and in three weeks, a definite change begins to occur. After six weeks, Margaret is just about back to normal. Margaret and Fred take the kids to Lollipop Land to make up for all the yelling.

Margaret is an excellent example of the psychological changes that occur when the body produces excessive levels of thyroid hormone. Some of these changes are:

- Increased excitability
- An emotional roller coaster of moods
- Outbursts of anger for no reason
- Crying spells
- A tendency to get easily distracted
- A very short attention span

Years ago, doctors often saw severe and longstanding cases of hyperthyroidism — patients with huge thyroid glands who were visibly shaky and nervous, unable to sit still for more than a few moments. That very rarely happens now, because the condition is usually diagnosed earlier, but rare cases of severe, prolonged hyperthyroidism may result in hallucinations, both in vision and hearing.

When hyperthyroidism affects elderly people (which I define as anyone older than I am), the condition may actually look like hypothyroidism. An elderly patient with hyperthyroidism may feel sad and depressed, apathetic, and withdrawn from society. I explain how thyroid problems affect the elderly in Chapter 18.

The treatments for hyperthyroidism, which I describe in Chapter 6, are very effective in reversing all the mental symptoms and physical symptoms, particularly in younger people who often get the disease.

Fighting Depression

Depression may be a symptom of a lack of thyroid hormone. On the other hand, thyroid hormone may help in the treatment of depression, even when tests indicate that the patient has enough thyroid hormone. The following sections explain the role that thyroid hormone plays in depression.

Determining if the thyroid is causing depression

Depression is a prominent symptom of thyroid disease, especially hypothyroidism. Therefore, when someone is diagnosed with depression, it's important to determine whether a thyroid disease is the cause.

Studies have shown that most depressed people do not have hypothyroidism. However, the condition may be found in a mild form in as many as 20 percent of depressed people, more often in women than in men. If hypothyroidism is diagnosed, a doctor should determine whether the patient is taking a drug for treatment of depression that could actually be causing hypothyroidism (see Chapter 10). Two such drugs are lithium and carbamazepine.

If a drug is responsible for hypothyroidism, there are two options. The patient can be taken off the drug, in which case its contribution to the depression will disappear, but the patient may still be depressed for other reasons. Alternately, the patient can be treated with thyroid hormone if the doctor feels that the drug is helping the depression a great deal and no substitute exists.

Finding a thyroid specialist

If you feel that you need the help of a specialist in thyroid diseases, there are many ways that you can find one. The first step is to ask your general doctor to recommend one to you. If your doctor refuses to do so, or if you are not happy with his or her choice, there are many alternatives:

✔ You can ask the referral service of a nearby hospital for the name of a thyroid specialist who is Board Certified in Endocrinology. This ensures that you will get a specialist and not a general doctor who likes to take care of thyroid cases.

✔ You can go on the Web to the site of the American Association of Clinical Endocrinologists at www.aace.com. On the first page under "Services," click on "Find an Endocrinologist." The page that comes up requires you to fill in the city and state where you want your doctor and open the box to "Select a Specialty." Here you can choose "Thyroid Dysfunction." Once you have filled in the boxes appropriately, click on "I Need A Doctor." You will be given a list of members of the AACE in your area who specialize in thyroid disease.

✔ Go to the Web site of the American Thyroid Association at www.thyroid.org. Although there are no lists of specialists, the site does tell you how to contact this organization of thyroid scientists so that you can find a member in your area to whom you might go for help.

If you are being treated for depression and have not had thyroid function tests, ask your doctor to have them performed.

Using thyroid hormone to treat depression

Many doctors believe that there's a role for replacement thyroid hormone in the treatment of depression, even when no thyroid abnormality is found.

Given by itself, thyroid hormone does not seem to reverse depression in a patient who does not have a thyroid disease. However, when the thyroid hormone *triiodothyronine* (see Chapter 3) is given together with antidepressants, it can improve the effectiveness of the treatment. This is especially true when a patient is taking a class of drugs called *tricyclic antidepressants,* which have brand names like Elavil, Tofranil, Etrafon, Norpramin, and Sinequan. The thyroid hormone is particularly effective in turning people who do not respond to those drugs into responders. It also increases the effectiveness of those drugs when they do work.

When used to help treat depression in patients who do not have thyroid disease, the thyroid hormone can be stopped after a few weeks or months and the positive effect persists.

TSH, autoantibodies, and depression

Thyroid abnormalities are often associated with other chemical changes in the blood besides too much or too little thyroid hormone. A patient with hypothyroidism, for example, may have too much *thyroid-stimulating hormone (TSH)* or high levels of *thyroid autoantibodies,* both of which are explained in Chapter 3. Could these other chemical changes promote depression in some patients?

No correlation has been found to date between levels of these other chemical substances and depression. Patients may sometimes have high autoantibodies while their thyroid function is normal, in which case they don't experience thyroid-related depression. The level of TSH in the blood does not seem to impact depression either.

Current research indicates that the level of the thyroid hormones themselves affect mood, and the levels of these other substances do not.

Chapter 3

How the Thyroid Works

The thyroid is a unique organ or gland that affects every part of the body. It does so by making hormones and sending them into the bloodstream, which carries them to every other cell and organ. (*Hormones* are substances made in one organ and carried by body fluids to another organ, where they produce an effect.) These hormones perform many different functions depending upon the particular organ they are sent to.

In this chapter, I show you how to locate the thyroid. If you are really perceptive and your thyroid is a little on the larger side, you may even be able to feel it. I also describe for you the names of the various hormones that control the thyroid and that the thyroid produces. Because your body contains many organs that perform various functions, I explain what thyroid hormones do in each organ to make that organ work more efficiently.

This chapter also shows you how to recognize when the thyroid is abnormal in size and shape and what happens to the body when thyroid hormones are produced in too large or too small quantities.

If you read this whole chapter, you'll know so much about thyroid function that you'll never suffer from *hamburger hyperthyroidism,* a real disease that results from eating cuts of meat that include the thyroid gland of the cow.

By the time you finish this chapter, I expect that you will have a much greater appreciation for your thyroid gland. You might even take out a piece of paper and write "I love my thyroid" 100 times.

Locating the Thyroid

Have you ever seen one of those wonderful anatomy books where you can peel the layers away starting from the skin down to see all the inner structures of the body? If you did that with the neck, as soon as you peeled away the skin you would find a bony, V-shaped notch created by the connection of the inside edges of the collar bones. The tissue that surrounds the front and sides of the *trachea* (windpipe) between the V and your Adam's apple is the *thyroid gland.* It is shown in Figure 3-1 with some of the more important surrounding structures.

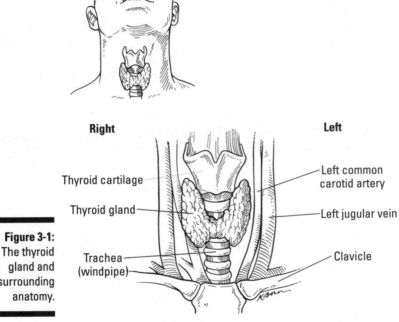

Right   **Left**

Thyroid cartilage

Thyroid gland

Trachea
(windpipe)

Left common
carotid artery

Left jugular vein

Clavicle

Figure 3-1:
The thyroid
gland and
surrounding
anatomy.

If you want to find your thyroid (without peeling away your skin), place your index finger at that bony notch below your Adam's apple and push your finger toward the back of your neck. If you then swallow, you may feel something push up against your finger. That is your thyroid gland.

In Figure 3-1, you can see that the thyroid has the shape of a butterfly. The wings of the butterfly are called the *left* and *right lobes* of the thyroid. Connecting the lobes is the *isthmus,* a narrow strip of tissue between the two larger parts. Sometimes you can see a third thyroid lobe called the *pyramidal lobe,* another narrow strip of thyroid tissue rising up from the isthmus.

When the thyroid is normal in size, it weighs between 10 and 20 grams. That would be between one-fiftieth and one-twenty-fifth of a pound — not terribly large considering everything it does. Each lobe of the thyroid is only about the size of your thumb. Even so, the thyroid is one of the largest hormone-producing glands in your body.

If you look at the thyroid under a microscope, you can see that it consists of rings of cells one cell deep with a clear center that contains the thyroid hormones. The rings are called *follicles* and are shown in Figure 3-2.

Producing Thyroid Hormones

The production of thyroid hormones actually begins in the brain, as shown in Figure 3-3. A structure called the *hypothalamus* produces a hormone called *thyrotrophin-releasing hormone* (TRH). This hormone is carried a short distance in the brain to the pituitary gland, where it promotes the release of *thyroid-stimulating hormone* (TSH).

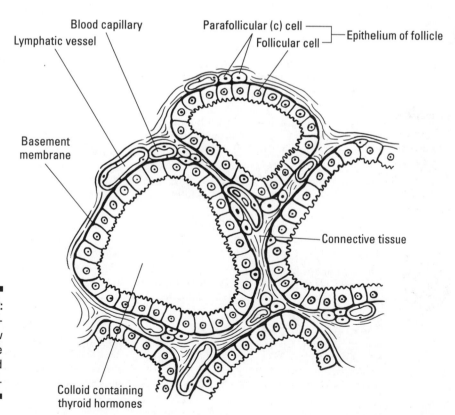

Blood capillary
Lymphatic vessel
Parafollicular (c) cell
Follicular cell
Epithelium of follicle
Basement membrane
Connective tissue
Colloid containing thyroid hormones

Figure 3-2:
A micro-scopic view of the thyroid gland.

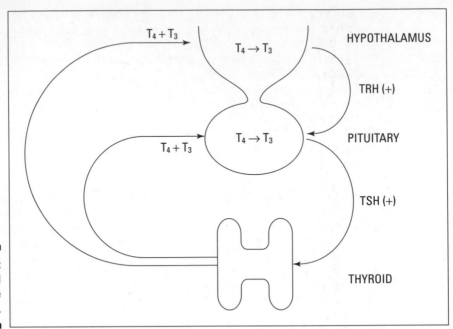

Figure 3-3:
Thyroid
hormone
production.

TSH leaves the pituitary gland and travels in the bloodstream to the thyroid, where it causes the production and release of two thyroid hormones: *thyroxine* (T4) and *triiodothyronine* (T3).

T3 is the active form of thyroid hormone. T4 is considered a *prohormone,* a much weaker chemical that gains its potency only after it is converted to T3. The conversion of T4 to T3 takes place in the many organs of the body (wherever thyroid hormones do their work), not just in the thyroid. The thyroid gland normally releases about 13 times as much T4 as T3. However, the body as a whole produces only about 3 times as much T4 as T3. This is because most (80 percent) of the T3 in the body comes from T4 that is converted in organs such as the liver, kidneys, and muscles. The thyroid gland itself releases only 20 percent of the T3 produced every day.

The statement in the previous paragraph has profound importance for the treatment of thyroid hormone deficiencies. Most patients with hypothyroidism (low thyroid function) are deficient in T3 and T4, but during treatment — when ingesting daily doses of replacement thyroid hormone — they receive only T4. Their bodies must get the T3 they need by converting the T4. Despite the conversion, these patients are still somewhat deficient in T3. I discuss this problem and possible solutions in Chapter 5.

Identifying the importance of iodine

Both thyroid hormones contain iodine. (T4 contains four parts of iodine, which make up 65 percent of its weight. T3 has three parts of iodine, which make up 58 percent of its weight.) This means that the thyroid gland must trap iodine to make the hormones. Because of this fact, we are able to study the workings of the thyroid by substituting radioactive iodine for regular iodine. Radioactive iodine can be detected and measured with a refined version of a Geiger counter (see Chapter 4) to perform a study called a *thyroid scan and uptake.*

Other organs, such as the breasts, the stomach, and the salivary glands, also trap iodine. However, no other organ in the human body besides the thyroid gland uses iodine for any important purpose. Thyroid hormones are the only significant chemicals that contain iodine.

Regulating thyroid hormones

When thyroid-stimulating hormone (TSH) reaches the thyroid, it prompts two reactions. First, it causes the release of existing thyroid hormone into the blood. Second, it prompts the production of more thyroid hormone, both T3 and T4, which collects in the space inside the follicles, awaiting future release. (If your TSH levels are elevated, it can also stimulate overall growth of your thyroid that can lead to an enlarged thyroid, called a *goiter.*)

Proteins that carry thyroid hormones

Three different proteins carry thyroid hormones. By far the most important is *thyroxine-binding globulin,* responsible for carrying 75 percent of the hormone in the blood. *Transthyretin,* which used to be called *thyroxine-binding prealbumin,* carries 20 percent of the thyroid hormones. *Thyroxine-binding albumin* carries the other 5 percent.

Exactly why proteins carry thyroid hormones is not clear. Among the theories is that by having so much thyroid hormone bound to proteins and therefore inactive, large changes in the thyroid gland's output of thyroid hormones will not result in large changes in thyroid activity. Another theory is that the combination of the hormone and the protein produces a large molecule, which cannot escape from the body through the urine, thus preserving iodine.

The released T3 and T4 circulate throughout the body, reaching, among other places, the pituitary gland. If the pituitary gland detects enough thyroid hormone, it continues to release the same amount of TSH. If thyroid hormone levels drop for any reason, the pituitary releases more TSH to stimulate the thyroid to make and release more thyroid hormone, if it can. If thyroid hormone is excessive, TSH release falls. (This is called the *negative feedback for TSH release.*)

In short, as thyroid hormone falls, TSH rises, and as thyroid hormone rises, TSH falls. Because T3, T4, and TSH can all be measured in the blood, it's simple to determine the state of your thyroid function (see Chapter 4).

As I mention earlier in the chapter, TSH is also regulated by the release of thyrotrophin-releasing hormone (TRH) from the hypothalamus. Between TRH and thyroid hormones, the level of TSH in the blood remains very stable throughout life, and abnormal levels usually mean some disease is present.

Moving thyroid hormones around

After T3 and T4 are released from the thyroid, they don't just travel loosely in the blood to their targets. Proteins in the bloodstream carry them. Because 99.97 percent of thyroid hormone is attached to proteins, only 0.03 percent floats freely in the bloodstream.

Only the *free* thyroid hormone can leave your blood and enter your cells. The rest is solidly bound to proteins and is not available to perform the actions of thyroid hormone. When a doctor measures the *total* thyroid hormone in your blood, she measures bound hormone along with the unbound hormone. If she only knows the total T4 amount in your blood, she needs to order a second test to determine the unbound T4 — the hormone that is free in your blood. This is important because many drugs and diseases alter the blood levels of thyroxine-binding proteins — the proteins that thyroid hormones bind to. If a drug like estrogen, for example, increases the amount of thyroxine-binding proteins in your body, your thyroid makes more thyroid hormone to bind to these proteins, keeping the unbound thyroid hormone constant and normal. Yet the results of a total T4 blood test will be elevated. Conversely, testosterone, the male hormone, causes a decrease in the thyroxine-binding proteins. If your testosterone level rises, your thyroid makes less thyroxine and a measurement of total T4 shows a decrease (while the unbound T4 again remains normal).

Understanding the Function of Thyroid Hormones

Thyroid hormones are active in just about every cell and organ of the body. They perform general functions that increase the efficiency of each organ's specific functions, whatever they may be. This section tells you all about those functions and explains what too much or too little of the hormone would do to a healthy person.

Many of these changes may be caused by other factors besides too little or too much thyroid hormone. For example, an infection can raise your body temperature just as too much thyroid hormone will. Also, if you have a condition like menopause that tends to be associated with dry skin, this symptom may predominate even if you have hyperthyroidism that tends to cause moist skin. The information here shows you what classic symptoms of thyroid problems look like, but each case can have individual variations.

General functions

In every cell, thyroid hormones cause that cell to make more *protein enzymes,* the chemicals that promote your metabolism. Think of your body as a machine. Adding extra thyroid hormone is like adding a richer fuel to it. The result is usually a revving up of the machine — like going from 2,000 revolutions per minute to 4,000 or more revolutions per minute, depending upon the amount of hormone added. Thus, when more thyroid hormone is present in your body, more chemical reactions are taking place.

Metabolism

The *basal metabolic rate* (BMR) is an overall measure of the amount of metabolism that is taking place in the body. Increased thyroid hormone may increase the BMR as much as 60 to 100 percent. Any machine that increases its activity heats up. Likewise, your body heats up with more thyroid hormone, and the result is a higher body temperature. At the other end, not enough thyroid hormone results in an abnormally low body temperature.

As more metabolism takes place, more of your food intake is burned for energy, so less is left to be stored. Your body detects the need for more energy and you get hungrier, but your faster metabolism usually more than offsets any increase in food intake. The net result is that you lose weight. However, when you take in too much extra food, you actually gain weight.

Muscle function

Your muscles need thyroid hormone for proper functioning, but too much is not a good thing. Too much thyroid hormone results in muscle wasting, as muscle tissue is consumed for energy. As you lose muscle, you become weaker. If too much thyroid hormone is present, the nerves going to the muscles also show increased excitability, resulting in increased reflexes and tremor in the muscles.

Many diet programs, recognizing that increased thyroid hormone results in weight loss, use thyroid hormones. An overabundance of thyroid hormone results in muscle loss, so the weight that you lose is not fat but muscle, the so-called lean tissue of the body. You do not want to lose lean tissue. Do not use thyroid hormone in an attempt to lose weight.

Energy sources

In addition to the protein found in muscle, thyroid hormone also affects the other sources of energy in the body, namely *carbohydrates* and *fats*. Carbohydrates are the main source of immediate energy in the body, so they get used up faster than normal when thyroid hormone levels rise, again resulting in more heat production. Fat is also used up faster than normal. The result is a lowering of the different kinds of fat in the body, namely *cholesterol* and *triglycerides*. On the other hand, when thyroid hormone levels drop, the fats accumulate in the liver and the level of cholesterol in the blood rises.

Because chemical reactions require vitamins, your need for vitamins increases when you have more thyroid hormone. Increased thyroid hormones cause a more rapid breakdown of the vitamins. Vitamins have little effect upon the thyroid gland itself, except for those that contain iodine (often in the form of kelp or seaweed). This iodine should be avoided when you are being treated for hyperthyroidism or have a condition like multinodular goiter (see Chapter 9) where the iodine may be used to make too much thyroid hormone.

Specific functions

Every organ in your body requires thyroid hormone to function normally. When that hormone is lacking, the organ tends to do less of its usual function. When too much thyroid hormone is present, the organ does more than it should. In this section, you find the most important changes brought on by abnormal amounts of thyroid hormone in the body. By no means is this discussion complete. That would require a large book by itself, and many of the changes that occur are too subtle to result in signs or symptoms that can be detected.

The heart

The heart needs T4 thyroid hormone for proper pumping. If not enough T4 is present, the heart slows down and its pumping action decreases. If T4 is severely lacking, heart failure can result. Conversely, when T4 levels rise, the heart rate is too rapid. The heart pumps out more blood at first, but if this increased pumping is allowed to go on too long, the end result may be decreased heart strength because excessive T4 causes muscle wasting. (The heart is made of muscle.)

Depending upon the level of your physical activity, your normal resting heart rate should be between 60 and 80. (If you are in good physical condition, your heart rate should be around 60.) People with too much T4 often have a heart rate of 120 or faster.

The lungs

As you increase your metabolism, you need more oxygen for the chemical reactions in your body to take place. Oxygen comes into the body through the lungs. Your respiration rate, normally about 16 times per minute, speeds up to bring in more oxygen. However, even an increased respiration rate may fail to provide the body with enough oxygen if the muscular diaphragm and chest muscles are wasting from excess T4.

The stomach and intestines

T4 is required for the muscles of the stomach and intestines to push food along for digestion and excretion. When not enough T4 is present, intestinal movement slows, as well as the absorption of food. The common complaint is constipation. On the other hand, too much T4 speeds up the bowels. Loose bowel movements, more frequent bowel movements, or diarrhea may be the result.

The skin, hair, and nails

The increase in blood flow with increased T4 is especially prominent in the skin. The skin often feels warm and perspiration may increase, so it also feels moist. When T4 levels fall, the skin often becomes dry and may scale. It feels cold to the touch. The nails cannot achieve their proper toughness without enough thyroid hormone and may break easily. The hair, likewise, is fragile, and excessive hair loss is a common complaint when not enough T4 is present.

The brain and cerebral functioning

Chapter 2 details the changes in mood that occur with too much or too little thyroid hormone. The person with excessive T4 may feel as if her brain is racing, which can result in extreme nervousness. She may feel anxious without knowing why and become worried about minor things. In extreme cases, the result may be paranoia. Not enough T4 can lead to mental dullness and depression.

Sexual functioning and menstruation

Thyroid hormone is needed for normal sexual function. Both men and women lose interest in sex when not enough T4 is present. They do not necessarily have increased interest in sex when T4 levels rise, because so many psychological and physical problems result from the increase.

The menstrual cycle depends on adequate T4 to proceed normally. Women with a lack of T4 may have trouble conceiving a baby. They tend to have increased menstrual flow and may become anemic (resulting from losing too much blood). Too much T4 often decreases the menstrual flow or causes missed periods.

The bones

Thyroid hormones help keep bone growth normal. When too little thyroid hormone is present in early life, the bones show delayed development and do not grow to their correct length. The result is a dwarf with short arms and legs and a larger trunk. If thyroid hormone is lacking after growth has stopped, the bones appear more dense than normal because of decreased bone turnover.

With an overabundance of thyroid hormone, whether it is due to taking too much thyroid hormone or inadequate treatment of hyperthyroidism, bone turnover and loss increases. The result may have the appearance of osteoporosis, the kind of bone loss that occurs in women after menopause. However, it rarely results in bone fractures if the increased thyroid hormone is controlled with treatment (because the bone loss stops).

Chapter 4

Testing Your Thyroid

These days, we take for granted our ability to precisely measure thyroid function. Yet only 60 years ago, measurements were so primitive that we depended more upon the physical and emotional state of the patient than the lab tests to make a diagnosis. This was unfortunate because the patients with obvious signs and symptoms are just the tip of a huge iceberg of thyroid abnormalities.

Today, the tests that measure thyroid function are getting more and more sensitive. Doctors can identify many people with *subclinical* thyroid disease (which means that its symptoms are not yet apparent to the patient or the doctor) that may be slowly damaging the patient and will become clinical sooner or later in any case. This is especially true in our aging population, whose symptoms of aging are so similar to those of mild hypothyroidism.

Although you cannot order the tests described in this chapter for yourself, this information can increase your understanding of what various tests involve and what their results mean. The information in this chapter can help you have better discussions with your doctor about your diagnosis.

Checking the Blood Levels of Thyroid Hormone

Numerous blood tests can be done to measure thyroid function, but the most accurate and sensitive tests for determining thyroid function are the *free thyroxine* (FT4) and the *thyroid-stimulating hormone* (TSH) tests, both of which are described in this section. (Free thyroxine is the tiny portion of thyroid hormone in the blood that is free to get into cells; see Chapter 3.) The vast majority of people are accurately diagnosed with these tests. If you're being screened for thyroid function and your doctor wants to order just one test to start, that test should be the TSH because of its accuracy and the fact that it's a simple blood test.

Many doctors practicing today learned about thyroid disease when only older tests were available, and they still use them. Just in case your doctor orders such tests, or in case you have copies of old test results that you want to understand, in this section I also explain how some of the older tests work (although the sooner they are dropped from the list of tests that labs will do, the better for patients).

Total thyroxine

The *total thyroxine* or *TT4 test* (sometimes called the *T4 immunoassay*) measures all the T4 thyroid hormone in a given quantity of blood. Most of the hormone measured is inactive because it is bound to protein (see Chapter 3). By itself, this test does not tell you how much thyroid activity is present. To give a more accurate picture of active thyroid hormone function, this test needs to be combined with a test that measures what percent of the total thyroxine is bound and what percent is free.

The total thyroxine test can also be deceiving because many drugs and clinical states raise the level of TT4 in your blood (because they raise the amount of thyroxine-binding protein in your system), yet they don't impact the amount of free thyroxine. Some of the drugs that can raise the level of TT4 in your blood include

- Estrogenic hormones taken for hormone replacement or birth control
- *Amiodarone,* a drug used for the heart
- Amphetamines
- Methadone

Some clinical states that can raise TT4 levels include

- High estrogen states, such as pregnancy
- Acute illness, such as AIDS or hepatitis
- Acute psychiatric problems

Conversely, some drugs and physical conditions tend to lower the results of a TT4 test (because they depress the amount of thyroxine-binding protein), *while not impacting the amount of free thyroxine.* The drugs that have this impact include

- *Androgens,* male hormones taken to build muscle
- *Steroids,* usually given to reduce inflammation
- *Nicotinic acid,* given to lower harmful blood fats
- Aspirin in high doses (more than 3,000 milligrams daily)

Physical conditions that can lower TT4 levels include

- Severe chronic illness such as kidney failure or liver failure
- Starvation

A normal range of TT4 would be 5 to 11 micrograms per deciliter of blood.

Different laboratories may use different techniques to perform the same test, resulting in slightly different normal values. Even when they use the same technique, there may be slight variations in the normal values from lab to lab since those values are derived from each lab's own group of people without thyroid disease.

If your doctor chooses to use the total thyroxine test to monitor your thyroid function, he or she must make certain that you aren't taking any of the drugs or experiencing any of the physical conditions listed in this section. In addition, your doctor must also order the next test, the resin T3 uptake, to get a complete picture.

Resin T3 uptake

The *resin T3 uptake* measures whether there are a lot of sites for T3 hormone (active thyroid hormone) to bind to on thyroxine-binding proteins. This occurs when the TT4 is low (and therefore taking up very few of the sites) or the binding protein levels are very high.

How the resin T3 uptake is done

When radioactive T3 or T4 is mixed with your blood in a test tube, it combines with the binding sites on the thyroxine-binding proteins. If your blood is then exposed to a substance called a *resin* that will bind the unbound T3 or T4, the resin can be measured for radioactivity. The result can be expressed as the percent of radioactivity found on the resin, compared to the original radioactivity that was added. The more binding sites that are open on your proteins, the lower the resin uptake result will be, and vice versa.

Anything that reduces the binding sites, thus causing a low TT4 measurement, leaves very few binding sites for any more thyroid hormone to bind to. If T3 is added to a sample of that blood, little T3 will be bound, leaving a lot of measurable free T3. The resin T3 uptake will be high. Anything that raises the binding sites, thus causing an increased TT4 level, also leaves a lot of binding sites available for added T3. The amount of free T3 measured will be low, giving a decreased resin T3 uptake. The usual result of a resin T3 uptake is 25 to 35 percent depending on the lab.

Free thyroxine index

As I indicate in the previous sections, the total thyroxine (TT4) test and the resin T3 uptake must be used together to be valuable. In the "Total thyroxine" section, I note several drugs and physical conditions that can alter the results of the TT4 test (and that also alter the resin T3 uptake results). The impact of such drugs and physical conditions always affects the TT4 and resin T3 uptake results in opposite directions: If the TT4 is depressed, then the resin T3 uptake is high; if the TT4 is elevated, the resin T3 uptake is low.

To determine a useful test result, doctors multiply the TT4 level by the resin T3 uptake. The result, called the *free thyroxine index,* is an indicator of thyroid function and usually falls between 1.25 and 3.85. A free thyroxine index below 1.25 indicates low thyroid function, and a result above 3.85 indicates increased thyroid function.

Even if you are taking one of the drugs or experiencing one of the physical conditions listed in the "Total thyroxine" section, the free thyroxine index should be within the normal range if your thyroid is functioning normally.

Free thyroxine (FT4)

The *free thyroxine* (FT4) test is the best way to measure the amount of free thyroid hormone in your blood. This test measures the 0.03 percent of T4 that is not bound to protein — the T4 that is free to interact with your cells (see Chapter 2). All the factors that can change the amount of total thyroxine in your system, such as the drugs and physical conditions listed earlier in the chapter, do not affect the amount of FT4 in your blood. Depending upon the test method that is used by the particular laboratory, the usual FT4 level is around 1 to 3 ng/dl (nanograms per deciliter).

The level of FT4 in your blood is high if you have hyperthyroidism and low if you have hypothyroidism. (As I explain in more detail in Chapter 6, in rare cases a patient with hyperthyroidism has too much T3 rather than too much T4 in her blood. In these rare instances, an FT4 test could come back normal or even low.)

The FT4 is not a perfect test, because there are certain conditions that make the FT4 level appear abnormal when the patient actually has normal thyroid function. Fortunately, these conditions are easily recognized. They include the following:

✔ Patients with severe chronic illness (not thyroid disease) may have slight decreases in FT4.

✔ People producing or eating large amounts of T3 have decreased FT4.

✔ The rare patient with resistance to T4 has high levels of FT4 yet is not hyperthyroid. This may be a hereditary condition.

✔ Patients on heparin to prevent blood clotting may have slight increases in FT4.

✔ Patients with acute illness may briefly have elevated FT4 as binding proteins suddenly fall.

Free triiodothyronine (FT3)

This test measures the free T3 hormone in the blood. This test is rarely necessary, except in the situation where a patient is hyperthyroid, yet the FT4 test result is normal. The usual level of FT3 is 0.25 to 0.65 ng/dl (nanograms per deciliter). A hyperthyroid patient has a high FT3 result. A hypothyroid patient has a low FT3 result.

Thyroid-stimulating hormone (TSH)

The *thyroid-stimulating hormone* (TSH) test is the most sensitive test of thyroid function in most circumstances. The TSH rises when the T4 level in the blood falls, and the TSH falls when the T4 rises (see Chapter 3). The assays used to measure TSH are the most accurate assays currently being done, so this is an excellent test to measure thyroid function. If you have hyperthyroidism, your TSH level is low (because TSH production is suppressed by the high level of T4 in your blood). If you have hypothyroidism, your TSH level is high (because your body is trying to stimulate the production of more T4). Always depending on the particular laboratory doing the test, the TSH is usually 0.5 to 5 mU/ml (microunits per milliliter).

Many different conditions can cause a reduction in the TSH level. A low TSH does not necessarily mean that you have hyperthyroidism. Some of the factors that can decrease your TSH include

✔ Excessive treatment with T3 or T4 hormone

✔ Thyroid nodules that make excessive T3 or T4 (see Chapter 6)

✔ The first trimester of pregnancy (A hormone called *chorionic gonadotrophin* is produced during the first trimester, which has TSH-like properties and stimulates the production of T4, thereby suppressing TSH.)

✔ The cancer *choriocarcinoma* or molar pregnancy, both of which are associated with the production of large amounts of the hormone chorionic gonadotrophin

✔ A pituitary tumor that destroys TSH-producing cells

✔ "Euthyroid" Grave's disease, where hyperthyroidism is present in the thyroid but the thyroid is not making levels of T4 that would be called excessive (see Chapter 5)

✔ Acute depression

Several conditions can cause an increase in your TSH level, even if your thyroid is not underactive. The following conditions have to be considered when a high TSH is found:

✔ A pituitary tumor involving the cells that make TSH

✔ Recovery from a severe illness

✔ Insufficient dietary iodine

✔ Resistance to the action of T4

✔ Failure of the adrenal gland to make adrenal hormone

✔ Psychiatric illness

Many of the conditions listed in this section are temporary, meaning that a patient's TSH level will return to normal if she just waits. Other conditions, such as a pituitary tumor, require action (in this case, the removal of the tumor) to restore the TSH to its normal level.

Sometimes a condition that suppresses production of TSH, such as hyperthyroidism, produces a low TSH level for some time even after you've returned to a normal metabolic state with treatment. The FT4 is normal, but the TSH remains low. This is one occasion when the TSH cannot be used as a reliable guide to thyroid function, so the FT4 is used instead.

After your doctor establishes a diagnosis for a thyroid problem, you may have repeated TSH tests during the course of your treatment to monitor your progress. If you are being treated for hyperthyroidism, however, repeated TSH tests may not be the most effective way to monitor progress, because your TSH may not recover for a long time after your metabolism returns to normal.

Taking Non-Hormonal Blood Tests

If you have thyroid disease, that does not necessarily mean that your thyroid is functioning too much or too little. For example, a patient who has thyroid inflammation or thyroid cancer could have normal levels of FT4 and the TSH. In this situation, blood tests other than those described in the previous section may be helpful in making the correct diagnosis. In this section, I help you understand when these tests are necessary and how you interpret their results.

Thyroid autoantibodies

Many thyroid conditions, which I explain in detail in later chapters, are called *autoimmune diseases* because they appear to result from the body rejecting its own tissue. If you look at diseased thyroid tissue under a microscope, it contains many of the same cells that would be found if a foreign invader were present in the body, such as if an organ were transplanted from one person to another.

The tissue, cell, or chemical that the body is trying to reject is called an *antigen.* The chemical (usually a protein) that the body manufactures to reject an antigen is called an *antibody.* When an antibody is directed against your own tissue, it is called an *autoantibody* (an antibody directed against yourself).

When you have an autoimmune thyroid disease, many autoantibodies are found in your body, but the two principal ones are called *antithyroglobulin autoantibody* and *antimicrosomal* (now called *thyroid peroxidase*) *autoantibody.* (Bet you can't say that three times fast.) Antiperoxidase autoantibodies are found more often than antithyroglobulin autoantibodies.

If your doctor wanted to confirm a diagnosis of autoimmune thyroid disease, he or she would order tests of your antithyroid autoantibodies and thyroid peroxidase autoantibodies. If either test returned at a level of over 100 international units per milliliter, the diagnosis would be confirmed.

These autoantibodies are found at the highest levels in patients with a condition called *Hashimoto's thyroiditis* (which I explain in Chapter 5), but they are also found in patients with *Graves' disease,* a form of hyperthyroidism (see Chapter 6). Autoantibodies are found at lower levels in up to 10 percent of normal people (the percentage increases with age). Some thyroid specialists believe that people with low levels of autoantibodies actually have subclinical (nonsymptomatic) thyroid disease. If this is true, the population with thyroid disease is far greater than previously thought.

If autoantibodies are not present in abnormal amounts, a diagnosis of Hashimoto's thyroiditis cannot be made.

Although each one is discussed in its own chapter in this book, the autoimmune diseases of the thyroid are actually different clinical presentations of the same underlying condition. The evidence for this is based upon the following facts:

- ✔ The thyroid tissue appears the same in the different conditions.

- ✔ Autoimmune thyroid disease runs in families.

- ✔ One person may pass through Graves' disease, Hashimoto's disease, and hypothyroidism at different times.

- ✔ The same types of autoantibodies are found in all three groups.

Some autoantibodies stimulate the thyroid, while others suppress the thyroid. At any given time, the condition of a patient with an autoimmune disease of the thyroid depends upon which group of antibodies is present at the highest levels. If there's more suppression than stimulation, the patient will have low thyroid function. If there's more stimulation than suppression, hyperthyroidism will result. The patient may start high, go back to normal, and end up low. Treatment sometimes does nothing more than speed up this process.

Finding autoantibodies may be a clue that thyroid disease will occur in the future. Relatives of people with autoimmune thyroid disease often have autoantibodies, and many of them develop thyroid disease at some point in life.

In up to 25 percent of patients, an autoimmune thyroid disease goes away after a time. A higher concentration of autoantibodies does not mean that a patient is sicker than someone who has a lower concentration. It may simply mean that the illness is less likely to go away.

One other autoantibody may be especially important in patients who have hyperthyroidism. This is the *thyroid-stimulating immunoglobulin* (TSI) that acts like TSH in stimulating the thyroid to make and release more hormones.

Theories explaining autoantibody production

Exactly why the body forms antibodies against its own tissue is not known, but there are several theories. Ordinarily, there are cells in the body that prevent production of antibodies against the self. It may be that people who form thyroid autoantibodies are deficient in those protective cells at some point early in life.

Another possibility is that the body is attacked at some point by a foreign invader (like a virus) that has antigens similar to those found in thyroid tissue. In making antibodies to fight the foreign antigens, the body makes antibodies that fight its own tissue as well.

Serum thyroglobulin

Thyroglobulin is the form in which thyroid hormones are packaged within the thyroid follicle (see Chapter 3). Thyroglobulin is found in the blood of normal individuals, but its levels are much higher when there is thyroid damage (for example, with cancer of the thyroid or inflammation of the thyroid). A normal level of thyroglobulin is between 3 and 42 nanograms per milliliter.

Doctors won't test the level of thyroglobulin in your blood for the purpose of making a diagnosis, because several different conditions cause elevations. Rather, this test is used to follow the course of a patient already diagnosed with a thyroid condition — especially a thyroid cancer patient, who will show an increase in thyroglobulin if the cancer grows and spreads. Immediately after surgery for thyroid cancer, the thyroglobulin level is very low, but if the cancer remains present and spreads, the thyroglobulin will increase.

Determining the Size, Shape, and Content of Your Thyroid

As I mention earlier in the chapter, free thyroxine (FT4) and thyroid-stimulating hormone (TSH) levels are normal in patients who have thyroid conditions where hormone activity is normal. Therefore, other types of tests may be necessary to gather information about the size, shape, and content of the thyroid gland. Even when a doctor has already diagnosed an abnormal thyroid activity, one or more of these studies may help to differentiate the causes. Each test is easy and painless and provides information that can be obtained in no other way.

Radioactive iodine uptake and scan

The thyroid concentrates iodine from the blood in order to make thyroid hormones (see Chapter 3). This fact has been used for decades to perform a study of the dynamic activity of the thyroid.

If radioactive iodine (in the form of a capsule that is swallowed) is given to a patient, a device like a Geiger counter can be passed over the thyroid in order to count the radioactivity. A normal thyroid appears like a butterfly (see Chapter 3) at the lower end of the neck. The counts of radioactivity are uniform throughout the thyroid. On paper, the counts are registered as dots. If the gland is normal, dots in every part of the gland are uniform and the picture on paper shows the shape and two-dimensional size of the gland.

When one thyroid nodule is overactive, most of the radioactive iodine concentrates in that nodule, giving it a darker appearance on paper. Because of this appearance, that spot of the thyroid is called a *hot nodule*. The rest of the gland is often suppressed and appears lighter; therefore it's said to be "cold." If the nodule itself does not concentrate as much iodine as the rest of the gland, it's called a *cold nodule*. Thyroid cancers are generally "cold," because cancerous parts of the thyroid do not produce thyroid hormone in the usual way. However, most cold nodules are not cancer.

In addition to showing the size and shape of the gland, a radioactive scan and uptake measures how active the thyroid is. When the thyroid is overactive, it takes up more iodine than normal. When it's underactive, it takes up less than normal. The maximum uptake of radioactivity usually occurs about 24 hours after swallowing the iodine. At this point, a normal thyroid has taken up between 5 and 25 percent of the administered dose of iodine. An overactive thyroid takes up 35 percent or more. Uptake between 25 and 35 percent is borderline.

Figure 4-1 shows the appearance of a normal thyroid scan and a scan that indicates hyperthyroidism. The second scan is much darker and shows a larger thyroid gland, consistent with the increased uptake and growth of the thyroid in hyperthyroidism.

Figure 4-1:
A normal thyroid and a hyperactive thyroid as shown in a radioactive iodine scan.

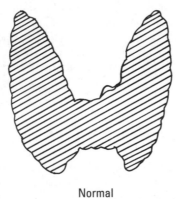

Normal

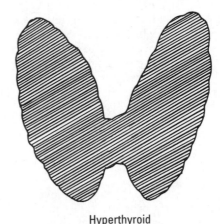

Hyperthyroid

There are a few situations that prevent obtaining a thyroid scan and uptake. If a patient takes in large amounts of iodine, that will both block iodine uptake by the thyroid and dilute the administered dose. If you take thyroid replacement hormone, that will block thyroid activity and reduce the uptake of radioactive iodine. Diseases, such as silent thyroiditis (see Chapter 12) where the iodine leaves the thyroid rapidly, also prevent a proper study.

In the past, the radioactive iodine scan and uptake was generally done to make a diagnosis of an overactive thyroid. This is not done as much anymore because the blood levels of T4 and TSH are usually definitive, along with the physical examination. The scan and uptake is used more often for a thyroid that's abnormal in shape to establish whether there are multiple nodules present (see Chapter 9) and to determine whether a nodule is overactive.

Thyroid ultrasound

The thyroid ultrasound, also known as an *echogram* or *sonogram,* is a study that uses sound to measure the size, shape, and consistency of thyroid tissue. There's no radiation used in an ultrasound study.

To get this test, you go to the testing facility and lie on your back on a table with your neck hyperextended. A gel is placed on the neck to assist in the transmission of the sound. A device called a *transducer* is passed over the area of the thyroid, sending out high-pitched sound waves that are reflected back by tissue and collected by a microphone. Tissue that contains water gives the best reflections, while solid tissue like bone gives poor reflections.

A thyroid ultrasound can measure the size of the thyroid or nodules very precisely. It can be used to follow treatment for an enlarged thyroid or nodule to see whether it's shrinking. It can tell the difference between a cyst that is filled with fluid (and is almost never a cancer) and a solid nodule, which may be a cancer.

This test is often used after a radioactive iodine scan detects an area that is cold. Is it cold because it contains no thyroid tissue, which is how a cyst appears, or is it cold because it contains cancerous thyroid tissue that is solid? The ultrasound can differentiate a cyst from a solid mass but cannot tell you whether the mass is cancer. (Most of the time, it is not cancer.)

Deciphering ultrasound

A beam of sound from an ultrasound device consists of high frequency sound waves. The frequency is far higher than anything the human ear can hear. Such a beam can be focused and directed just like a beam of light. When it strikes tissue, the tissue reflects a certain amount of sound back — the amount depends upon how dense the tissue is. Air hardly reflects back any of the beam at all, while tissue, which is made up of many layers and contains water, sends plenty of sound back. Different tissues absorb the sound differently, therefore reflecting the sound to a different extent. A cancer will appear differently on an ultrasound than normal thyroid tissue or a cyst filled with fluid. When the reflection returns, the sound energy is converted to light energy and electrical energy, which can be displayed on a cathode ray tube or made into a permanent record by exposing a film to the light energy.

Figure 4-2 shows a normal ultrasound study of the thyroid and one where there is a prominent nodule that is solid.

Fine needle aspiration biopsy (FNAB)

When a doctor has a question as to the type of tissue making up a growth on the thyroid, the *fine needle aspiration biopsy* (FNAB) may be the definitive test. It's just about painless and free of complications. A small needle is introduced into the growth, and tiny bits of tissue are removed by pulling back on the plunger to create a vacuum. The needle is moved to a few different places.

The tissue is sprayed on a fixative, stained, and examined for signs of cancer. Most of the time, cancer can be ruled out or in. Occasionally, the tissue won't provide a clear diagnosis, and the lobe (side) of the thyroid that contains the lump must be removed.

Normal ultrasound

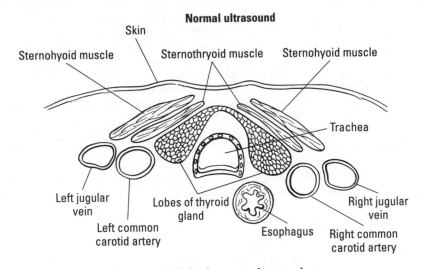

Skin

Sternohyoid muscle   Sternothryoid muscle   Sternohyoid muscle

Trachea

Left jugular vein

Lobes of thyroid gland

Right jugular vein

Left common carotid artery

Esophagus

Right common carotid artery

Nodule shown on ultrasound

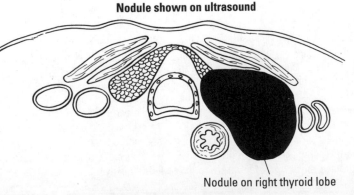

Figure 4-2: A normal ultrasound study (top) and an ultrasound that shows a solid nodule (bottom).

Nodule on right thyroid lobe

FNAB has saved thousands of patients from surgery and is often the first test performed to check for cancer, skipping the thyroid scan and the ultrasound. This is based on the Willie Sutton theory. Willie was a bank robber and was once asked why he robbed banks. His answer was "You go where the money is."

Part II
What's Wrong with My Thyroid?

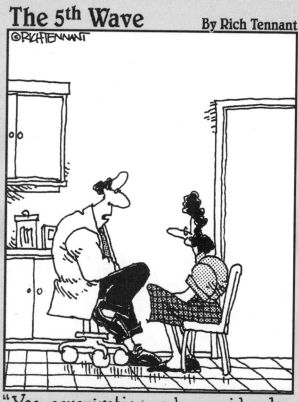

"Yes, perspiration and a rapid pulse could indicate hyperthyroidism. But the fact that these symptoms occur only when the pool boy is working in your backyard does raise some questions."

In this part . . .

The thyroid can be overactive or underactive. It can be too large or too small. It can be bumpy or smooth. The chapters in this part introduce you to all kinds of thyroid abnormalities. You discover how to recognize them and how to differentiate one from another. For those of you with thyroid disorders, I explain how they occur, which of the common signs and symptoms you have, how a particular disorder damages your body, and what you can do to cure it so no damage occurs.

Chapter 5

Diagnosing Decreased Thyroid Function

The most common form of thyroid disease throughout the world is *hypothyroidism* or low thyroid function (also known as *myxedema*). Hypothyroidism has numerous causes, but worldwide, iodine deficiency probably leads the list (see Chapter 12). In the United States and Europe, however, iodine deficiency is rare, and the leading cause of hypothyroidism is autoimmune thyroid disease.

In this chapter, I introduce you to the immensity of this problem, show you how hypothyroidism affects the body, and explain the proper treatment for the various forms of hypothyroidism. In the last few years, there have been some key changes in our understanding of hypothyroidism. I include that new information here so you can be up-to-date when you talk with your doctor about symptoms and treatment.

Living with Autoimmune Thyroiditis

Stacy Dummy, a 46-year-old woman, is the cousin of Sarah and Margaret Dummy, whom you meet in Chapter 2. She has generally been healthy but recently noticed some swelling in the lower part of her neck. The swelling seemed to develop very slowly, and she did not notice it until she tried to button a collar over her neck. Other than the swelling, she has really not had any physical problems. She is not gaining weight. She sleeps well at night and is not overly tired. She is not feeling unusually hot or cold. Her appetite is normal, as are her bowel movements. She has no discomfort associated with the growth in her neck.

Stacy's cousin Sarah, who was recently diagnosed with hypothyroidism, tells Stacy that she knows a good thyroid specialist who told her that other members of her family may have thyroid disease. Stacy goes to see Dr. Rubin, who examines her and finds that her thyroid gland is twice as large as normal. He finds no other significant abnormalities. He sends Stacy to the laboratory for two tests — a thyroid-stimulating hormone (TSH) test and a free thyroxine (FT4) test — both of which return within the normal range (see Chapter 4). Because of his clinical suspicion, Dr. Rubin also obtains thyroid autoantibody studies. These are very elevated, particularly the *thyroid peroxidase* autoantibodies, but also the *antithyroglobulin* autoantibodies (see Chapter 4).

Dr. Rubin tells Stacy that she has a condition called *chronic thyroiditis*. He tells her that treatment at this time is optional. If she is unhappy with the tissue sticking out on her neck, she can take thyroid hormone and it will shrink. If not, she need only return in six months or a year to check to see whether the disease has progressed to hypothyroidism.

Stacy's condition is a typical illustration of chronic thyroiditis, which is also called *Hashimoto's thyroiditis* or *autoimmune thyroiditis*. She is free of symptoms at this stage, and the only abnormality is a *goiter,* an enlargement of the thyroid. The blood tests that reflect thyroid function are normal. The high levels of thyroid autoantibodies in her system determine the diagnosis.

The extent of the problem

Most studies indicate that 10 percent of the world's population tests positive for thyroid autoantibodies (see Chapter 4). If the U.S. has a population of approximately 275 million people, about 27.5 million of them will test positive. Many experts (including me) believe that all these people have chronic thyroiditis. The vast majority will never be bothered by it.

Only about 1 in 1,000 of people who test positive for thyroid autoantibodies develop symptomatic chronic thyroiditis, which means that about 27,500 new cases occur in the United States each year. A woman is 20 times more likely to have symptomatic chronic thyroiditis than a man. The typical patient is 30 to 50 years old, but chronic thyroiditis is also found in children.

Chronic thyroiditis is a familial disease that is usually transmitted from mother to daughter. Even members of the family who show no symptoms often have thyroid autoantibodies in their blood (especially the females). They may develop hypothyroidism later on.

Symptoms of autoimmune thyroiditis

Some people with chronic thyroiditis do have symptoms, even when their thyroid function tests are normal. In addition to neck swelling, symptoms include

- ✔ Pain in the neck (which is unusual)
- ✔ Chest pain (which occurs in about 25 percent of patients)
- ✔ Trouble swallowing or a sensation of fullness in the neck
- ✔ Transient symptoms of hyperthyroidism (see Chapter 6) — but blood tests are not normal when this occurs

Approach to treatment

Being so benign, chronic thyroiditis that has not progressed to hypothyroidism is usually not treated. If you have neck pain because of chronic thyroiditis, aspirin will generally control it. If the swelling in your neck is unsightly or you have difficulty swallowing, your doctor will prescribe thyroid hormone to block the production of thyroid-stimulating hormone (TSH). Your thyroid gland will then shrink. Usually, it's a good idea to stop the hormone treatment at some later date, because up to one-quarter of patients with this condition have a remission and no longer need thyroid treatment.

If you experience transient symptoms of hyperthyroidism as a result of chronic thyroiditis, these usually require no treatment either. The symptoms usually last a few weeks, and then you return to normal. In especially severe cases, drugs that block the action of thyroid hormones (see Chapter 6) can be used.

Identifying Hypothyroidism

ANECDOTE

Karen Dummy is Stacy's younger sister. Over the last few years, she has noticed the gradual enlargement of her neck — a symptom similar to the one Stacy experienced. But Karen has had a number of other problems as well. She has gained a few pounds, and her legs appear swollen but do not retain an indentation when she presses on them. She feels cold when her husband feels comfortable and is constantly asking for more heat. Her skin is dry and her nails are brittle. She has dry hair and notices that she is losing more hair than before. The outer third of her eyelashes seems to have disappeared. She used to love to sing in choir, but her voice has become husky lately. She has trouble seeing to drive at night and notices trouble hearing as well.

Dr. Rubin, who is rapidly becoming the Dummy family doctor, examines her in his office. He finds that, in addition to all the symptoms Karen explains to him, she also has a slow pulse and an enlarged thyroid gland. He sends her for thyroid function tests (TSH and FT4) as well as thyroid autoantibody tests.

Karen's tests show that she has a low FT4 and a high TSH. Her autoantibody levels are elevated. Dr. Rubin makes a diagnosis of hypothyroidism due to chronic thyroiditis. He starts her on thyroid hormone replacement. Within six weeks, Karen is her old self. Full of gratitude, she puts Dr. Rubin in her will.

Signs and symptoms of hypothyroidism

Karen illustrates the classic signs and symptoms of hypothyroidism. The signs, including some that Karen did not show, are

- A slow pulse and enlarged heart
- An enlarged thyroid *(goiter),* unless prior removal of the thyroid gland is the cause of hypothyroidism
- Dry, cool skin that is puffy, pale, and yellowish
- White patches of skin where pigment is lost (a condition called *vitiligo*)
- Brittle nails and dry, brittle hair that tends to fall out excessively
- Swelling that does not retain an indentation, especially of the legs
- Hoarseness and slow speech with a thickened tongue
- An expressionless face
- Slow reflexes

Patients with hypothyroidism complain of many different symptoms, and each patient has unique complaints. Among the most common are

- Intolerance to cold
- Tiredness and a need to sleep
- Weakness
- Pain and stiffness in the joints and muscles
- Constipation
- Increased menstrual flow
- Trouble hearing and a ringing in the ears
- Trouble seeing at night

The physician who sees a patient with these signs and symptoms will obtain several tests to confirm the diagnosis. The two tests essential to the diagnosis are

  ✔ A free thyroxine (FT4) level that is lower than normal

  ✔ A thyroid-stimulating hormone (TSH) level that is higher than normal

Other tests that support the diagnosis include

  ✔ A mild anemia (decrease in red blood cells)

  ✔ An increased cholesterol count

  ✔ Elevated levels of thyroid autoantibodies (if the patient has autoimmune hypothyroidism)

  ✔ A blood glucose level that is lower than normal

After the diagnosis of hypothyroidism is made, the various causes of this condition need to be checked, because many of them are reversible without treating the thyroid directly.

Confusing conditions

The signs and symptoms of hypothyroidism are fairly nonspecific and can easily be confused with signs and symptoms of other common conditions. The three major sources of confusion are menopause, normal aging, and stress. All three are common occurrences for women, and men experience at least two out of the three (some people are now arguing that such a thing as male menopause exists). You can see how a person with low thyroid function could easily neglect to check for that condition. This is a major reason why doctors, including me, advise routine thyroid testing starting at age 35 and continuing every 5 years thereafter.

Pinpointing the Causes of Hypothyroidism

The two most common causes of hypothyroidism are iodine deficiency and chronic thyroiditis. Iodine deficiency is rare in the United States and Europe but very common throughout the rest of the world. I discuss this problem in detail in Chapter 12. As I discuss earlier in the chapter, chronic thyroiditis is an inherited condition that is diagnosed by checking the levels of thyroid autoantibodies in the blood.

In addition to these two causes, there are many other reasons that people become hypothyroid. The causes detailed in the following sections should be ruled out before your doctor starts treating your condition with thyroid hormone replacement.

Removal of the thyroid

If your thyroid has been removed because of cancer or an infection, or in the course of treatment for hyperthyroidism (see Chapter 6), you will usually become hypothyroid. Only if some tissue is left behind will the thyroid possibly continue to function.

Absence of brain hormones

Anything that destroys the *hypothalamus* (the part of the brain that secretes *thyrotrophin-releasing hormone*) or the *pituitary gland* at the base of the brain (which secretes thyroid-stimulating hormone) will produce *central hypothyroidism* — hypothyroidism originating in the control center of the body, the brain. A trauma, infection, or infiltration (a replacement of brain tissue with other tissue, which can occur when a patient has cancer) could cause this type of destruction. The same result can occur if the pituitary is involved with a destructive lesion that prevents the production and release of TSH, such as radiation treatment to the area of the pituitary gland.

If hypothyroidism is caused by a problem with the hypothalamus or pituitary, some of the signs and symptoms associated with chronic (autoimmune) thyroiditis will not be found. In particular, hoarseness and a thickened tongue occur in autoimmune hypothyroidism but not in hypothyroidism associated with a lack of brain hormones. In addition, the thyroid is not usually enlarged in this instance, because TSH is not stimulating it. Also, the patient's hair and the skin are not coarse in this situation (but they are if the patient has autoimmune hypothyroidism).

Symptoms that result from a lack of other pituitary hormones also help to differentiate central hypothyroidism from failure of the thyroid gland. These include fine wrinkling of the skin of the face and a more pronounced loss of underarm, pubic, and facial hair.

Foods that cause hypothyroidism

Many common foods can cause hypothyroidism if you eat them in sufficient quantities, especially if you have an iodine deficiency. These foods are called *goitrogens* because they can trigger the enlargement of the thyroid (a goiter) as well as hypothyroidism. They block the conversion of T4 hormone to T3, the active form of thyroid hormone (see Chapter 3). Among the more common foods that cause this condition are

- Almond seeds
- Brussels sprouts
- Cabbage
- Cauliflower
- Corn
- Kale
- Turnips

If your condition is caused by consuming these foods, simply removing them from your diet will cure your hypothyroidism. It takes between three and six weeks for your thyroid to return to normal after you stop eating these foods.

Drugs that cause hypothyroidism

Many different medications cause hypothyroidism in the same way as the goitrogens listed in the previous section: They block the conversion of T4 to T3. The drugs you are most likely to run into include

- Adrenal steroids like prednisone and hydrocortisone, which treat inflammation
- Amiodarone, a heart drug
- Antithyroid drugs like propylthiouricil and methimazole (see Chapter 6)
- Lithium, for psychiatric treatment
- Propranolol, a beta blocker (see Chapter 6)

Coexisting autoimmune diseases

Occasionally, a patient with autoimmune thyroid disease has other autoimmune diseases, many of which involve other glands of the body. For example, diabetes mellitus type 1 sometimes occurs together with autoimmune thyroid disease. The cause is the autoimmune destruction of the insulin-producing cells of the pancreas. Another example is Addison's disease, the autoimmune destruction of the adrenal gland. Addison's disease is associated with severe fatigue and low blood pressure and is especially important to identify, because giving thyroid hormone without adrenal hormone to such a patient could be dangerous.

Autoimmune destruction of the ovaries in women or the testicles in men may also occur when a patient has autoimmune thyroiditis. The result for women is failure to menstruate, and for men it is infertility and impotency.

Another gland that may be affected by autoimmune disease is the *parathyroid* (which actually consists of four parathyroid glands) sitting behind the thyroid in the neck. Loss of parathyroid function results in low blood calcium and the possibility of severe muscle spasms and psychological changes.

Some autoimmune diseases that affect the joints of the body are found together with autoimmune thyroiditis. Rheumatoid arthritis is the most common example, but other diseases with names like *Sjogren's syndrome* and *systemic lupus erythematosis* are also diagnosed.

Lastly, be aware of a blood disease called *pernicious anemia,* an autoimmune disease that accompanies autoimmune thyroiditis on occasion. In this condition, cells of the stomach that produce acid are destroyed by autoimmunity. The patient is unable to absorb vitamin B12 and develops an anemia along with symptoms in the nervous system.

On occasion, when these diseases occur together, treatment of one of them treats the other at the same time. For example, treating the hypothyroidism with thyroid hormone may greatly improve the diabetes.

Diagnosing Severe Hypothyroidism

Hypothyroidism is rarely seen in its severest form in the United States, but if the disease is left untreated and total thyroid failure occurs, the patient may die. The clinical picture that develops is one of extreme worsening of the signs and symptoms described earlier in the chapter. The skin becomes extremely dry and coarse, and the patient's hair falls out. She (or he) may lose all her eyelashes, and her body temperature may fall to a low level. The patient is less and less active and may lapse into a coma called *myxedema coma* that can last for many days until she dies of heart failure or infection. (The infection or heart disease may precipitate the myxedema coma in the first place in an elderly person with very low thyroid function.)

Because such a patient may not be taking in food or, if she is, the food is absorbed extremely slowly, treatment may require injections of thyroid hormones (described in the next section).

Treating Hypothyroidism

The treatment of hypothyroidism, once thought to be very complicated, is now fairly simple after a diagnosis is made. However, a number of newer thoughts on the subject are worth considering as you and your doctor discuss treatment.

Taking the right hormones

Patients with hypothyroidism caused by chronic thyroiditis or removal of the thyroid take daily thyroid hormone replacement pills.

The first treatment to replace absent thyroid hormone came from the thyroids of animals and was called *desiccated thyroid*. For many decades, it was the only treatment available.

When it became possible to make T4 hormone in the laboratory, T4 (also called *L-thyroxine*) replaced desiccated thyroid. This change was made for several reasons. First, the amount of hormone in a given animal's thyroid differed from animal to animal, so the dose delivered could never be standardized. Second, desiccated thyroid contained both T4 and T3 in amounts that were significantly different from the way it is secreted by the normal thyroid gland (see Chapter 3).

For many years, doctors suspected that generic forms of thyroid hormone replacement pills did not consistently provide a known level of the hormone, so doctors recommended brand name products. Recent studies show that generic thyroid hormone has the same potency as brand name thyroid hormone and is, of course, much cheaper.

Because 80 percent of the T3 thyroid hormone in your body comes from the conversion of T4 into T3 (at sites other than the thyroid), doctors used to believe that T4 could be given alone and the body would take care of producing the T3 it needs. But recent studies have not confirmed this to be true. When the human thyroid releases thyroid hormone, about 10 percent is T3 (and the rest is T4). In studies, hypothyroid patients who were given a mixture of T3 and T4 replacement hormone felt consistently better than patients given T4 alone.

Almost all people in the world who are currently receiving replacement thyroid hormone to treat hypothyroidism are taking T4 alone. In the future, treatment will consist of a mixture of T4 and T3 that approximates the secretion of these hormones by the thyroid gland. If you are receiving T4 and still do not feel right, ask your doctor if you can try a combination of T3 and T4.

If the cause of your hypothyroidism is something other than autoimmune failure of the thyroid or removal of the thyroid, that cause must be dealt with along with replacing the thyroid hormone that is deficient. For example, if you have a pituitary tumor that is responsible for a loss of TSH, the tumor must be treated, and other hormones need to be replaced in addition to thyroid hormones. If your hypothyroidism is caused by a drug or food, removal of that drug or food usually cures the condition. Sometimes the drug cannot be stopped, in which case thyroid hormone replacement is given to alleviate the hypothyroidism.

Getting the right amount

The amount of thyroid hormone that you receive is determined by doing a TSH test (assuming that central hypothyroidism is not the diagnosis). The normal blood level of TSH is 0.5 to 5 uU/ml in most laboratories.

Keep in mind that some doctors question whether this actually is the normal range for TSH. We know that 10 percent of the population tests positive for thyroid autoantibodies and probably has autoimmune thyroid disease. Most of these people are not given the diagnosis of hypothyroidism. When a laboratory creates a normal range, it tests several hundred or more people who are considered free of thyroid disease, usually because they have no signs or symptoms. The laboratory measures their TSH and states that "this is the range for TSH in the normal population." Are they really measuring a normal population when one of every ten people tested may have a subclinical thyroid disease?

In my practice, I have had several patients who did not feel normal with a TSH between 3 and 5. I have given these patients enough thyroid hormone to lower the TSH to under 3 with gratifying results. I believe that future studies will indicate that the normal range for TSH is more like 0.5 to 2.5.

If you are being treated for hypothyroidism and do not feel right on your current dose of replacement thyroid hormone, ask your doctor to check your TSH. If it is above 3, ask the doctor to prescribe more thyroid hormone to lower it below 3.

Another important point is that hypothyroidism is not necessarily permanent. Up to 25 percent of patients with autoimmune hypothyroidism may return to normal thyroid function at a later date. The reason is that the autoantibodies that block the action of TSH may decline over time.

If you have been treated for several years for autoimmune hypothyroidism, ask your doctor if you can stop the thyroid hormone replacement for four to six weeks to see whether your TSH will remain low. (Do not stop taking your hormone replacement without your doctor's supervision.)

On the other hand, a thyroid gland that is failing due to autoimmune thyroiditis goes through several levels of failure. At first, you may need little thyroid hormone to replace what you are missing. With time, more of your thyroid tissue may fail or the antibodies that block TSH may increase, and you will need more. It is important that you see your doctor on a regular basis to be checked for this increasing (or decreasing) failure of the thyroid.

After your thyroid function stabilizes, see your physician every six months or every year to have your TSH level checked and your dosage of thyroid hormone altered if necessary. These checkups are important because you may not feel different clinically even if your thyroid function gradually declines.

Testing hormone levels

It takes about four weeks for a change in your dose of replacement thyroid hormone to make a difference in your lab tests. If your dose is being changed, you should be retested about that often to make sure that you are on the correct dose.

Chapter 6

Taming the Hyperactive Thyroid

In This Chapter
▶ Recognizing the symptoms of hyperthyroidism
▶ Linking hyperthyroidism and Graves' disease
▶ Deciding on treatment
▶ Battling severe hyperthyroidism

*H*yperthyroidism refers to the excessive production of thyroid hormones, which leads to many signs and symptoms that suggest a patient's body is, in effect, speeding up.

Hyperthyroidism is fairly common. Each year, about 100 new cases are diagnosed per 100,000 people. That adds up to more than 275,000 new cases in the United States every year, because the U.S. population is at least 275 million.

Most people with hyperthyroidism (about 80 percent) have an autoimmune disorder called *Graves' disease,* which I discuss in detail in this chapter. In addition to causing signs and symptoms of hyperthyroidism, Graves' disease also causes eye disease and skin disease. These abnormalities are bound together by the fact that they are all the result of autoimmunity. (See Chapter 4 for a discussion of "Thyroid autoantibodies.") In some circumstances, a patient has hyperthyroidism but no eye disease or skin disease, and blood tests show no evidence of autoimmunity. These patients do not have an autoimmune disorder, but the medical picture produced by their hyperthyroid state is the same as if they had Graves'.

In this chapter, I show you how to recognize hyperthyroidism, what the treatment options are, and what possible complications may occur as a result of the treatment or the disease itself. You also discover how I would treat you if you came to me with Graves' disease.

Many people believe that if you have hyperthyroidism, you're lucky because it makes weight control or weight loss easier. By the time you finish this chapter, I hope you'll realize why that thinking is flawed.

Picturing Hyperthyroidism

Tami Dummy is the mother of Stacy and Karen, who have recently been diagnosed with autoimmune thyroiditis and hypothyroidism, respectively (see Chapter 5). Tami has always been a very active person, but lately she has noticed a lot of things wrong with her, and they are getting worse.

Tami feels warm all the time, and her skin is moist. A few months ago, she lost some weight without trying and was delighted, but the weight loss has continued despite the fact that she has a really strong appetite and is eating more than usual. She often feels her heart racing, which makes her very nervous. She notices that her hands shake when she just sits quietly. She goes to the bathroom more frequently than usual, both to urinate and to move her bowels.

The changes in Tami are not lost on her husband, Patrick, or her daughters. They notice that she is constantly staring at them, though when they question her, she denies it. Patrick, in the course of giving her a massage, notices a bump on the front of her neck that was not there before. Tami's family insists that she see their favorite doctor, none other than (did you guess?) Dr. Rubin.

Dr. Rubin asks a number of questions and does a physical examination. He discovers that Tami's thyroid is enlarged, and he finds a skin abnormality on her lower legs. He tells the family that Tami almost certainly has hyperthyroidism due to Graves' disease. The final diagnosis requires only some confirmatory blood tests, and the outcome of those tests is so certain that Dr. Rubin gives Tami a prescription for antithyroid pills at the first office visit.

The tests confirm the diagnosis. Tami immediately starts taking a pill three times a day. By the end of three weeks, she feels better, and after eight weeks, she is her old self. She is a bit disappointed when the pounds start coming back on, but she feels so good that she returns to her health club and sheds several of them in no time. Patrick is, of course, delighted to have his wife back at moderate instead of high speed. He has been wanting to go to the Oregon Shakespeare Festival, and he knew that she would not sit through a play in her previous condition.

Listing the Signs and Symptoms of Hyperthyroidism

Hyperthyroidism, whether caused by Graves' disease or another condition, produces consistent signs and symptoms that affect every part of your body.

The major abnormalities are described in the following sections, grouped according to the organ system of the body that is affected.

The body generally

Hyperthyroidism can cause your body temperature to be persistently high. You may lose weight despite an increased appetite. The weight loss is due to the loss of lean body tissue like muscle, not due to a loss of fat. In rare cases, a patient gains weight because she is eating so many calories. Hyperthyroidism can cause you to feel weak. You may feel lymph glands all over your body, because Graves' disease is an autoimmune disease and the lymph system is a key player in autoimmunity. Your tonsils, which are part of the lymph system, are also enlarged.

There are other possible reasons for the enlargement of lymph glands that are more serious than Graves' disease, so if you experience this, see your doctor.

The thyroid

When Graves' disease is the cause of hyperthyroidism, your thyroid is enlarged in a symmetrical way and the entire gland is firm. When a single overactive *nodule* (a bump on your thyroid) is to blame for hyperthyroidism, that nodule is large, but it often causes the rest of the gland to shrink. (See Chapter 7 for a discussion of nodules.) When a multinodular goiter is responsible (see Chapter 9), you can feel many lumps and bumps on your thyroid.

If you put your hand over an enlarged thyroid, you can often feel a buzz that is called a *thrill* and results from the great increase in blood flow in the overactive thyroid. You can hear the thrill with a stethoscope; the sound is called a *bruit.*

The skin and hair

Hyperthyroidism can cause your hands to feel warm and moist, and they may appear red. You may experience a loss of skin pigmentation (a condition called *vitiligo*) in places, which is another sign of autoimmunity. Other areas of your skin may appear darker. Your hair may be fine, straight, and unable to hold a curl.

The heart

Hyperthyroidism can cause a rapid pulse, which you feel as heart palpitations. The first sign of Graves' disease is sometimes *atrial fibrillation,* an irregular heart rhythm. If a patient is older and already has heart disease, hyperthyroidism can induce heart failure, or heart pain (angina) may appear or be made worse because the heart beats too rapidly. You may experience shortness of breath.

The nervous system and muscles

If you have hyperthyroidism, your fingers have a fine tremor when you hold your hands out. The loss of muscle tissue leads to weakness. Your reflexes are increased; some patients can't sit still. The mental changes associated with hyperthyroidism are discussed in Chapter 2. Basically, if you are hyperthyroid, most likely you're nervous, you don't sleep as much as you used to, and you have rapidly changing emotions, from exhilaration to depression.

The reproductive system

Hyperthyroidism can cause a decrease in fertility because it interferes with ovulation. Menstrual flow is decreased as well and may cease.

The stomach and intestines

If you are hyperthyroid, food moves more quickly through your intestines than it used to, and you have more frequent bowel movements or even diarrhea. You may experience nausea and vomiting.

The urinary system

As more blood flows, your kidneys filter more, and more urine is produced so you go to the bathroom more frequently. In turn, you feel more thirsty than usual.

The eyes

Any form of hyperthyroidism results in reversible changes to the eyes. Your upper eyelids may be pulled up higher so more of the white above the pupil is seen, which makes it appear as if you're staring and pop-eyed. When you are asked to look down, your upper eyelid may not follow your eye, which exposes even more white. This is called *lid lag*.

Graves' disease can cause more serious eye problems, which I discuss later in the chapter.

Confirming a Diagnosis of Hyperthyroidism

The signs and symptoms described in the previous section usually lead to a conclusive diagnosis of hyperthyroidism, which is confirmed by blood tests. Among the lab findings that can lead to a diagnosis, the following are most important:

- ✔ The levels of free T4 and free T3 (thyroid hormones) in your blood are elevated, and the thyroid-stimulating hormone (TSH) level is suppressed (see Chapter 4). The definitive tests for hyperthyroidism are the TSH and the free T4.

- ✔ If Graves' disease is the cause of hyperthyroidism, the levels of peroxidase autoantibody and antithyroglobulin autoantibody are elevated (see Chapter 4).

- ✔ Your blood glucose (sugar) level is elevated because your body is absorbing food so rapidly.

- ✔ You may have insulin resistance, and diabetes may be found or made worse if it's already present. (Diabetes improves after the hyperthyroidism is treated.)

- ✔ Blood tests of your liver function (such as the alkaline phosphatase and bilirubin levels in the blood) may be elevated.

- ✔ Blood tests for cholesterol and other fats may be lower than normal.

Determining Whether Graves' Disease Is the Culprit

Most cases of hyperthyroidism result from Graves' disease, an autoimmune condition. Graves' disease is most common in women; it occurs 10 to 20 times more often in women than in men. Symptoms tend to start between the ages of 30 and 60, but they can occur at any age. Graves' disease consists of any one or all of three parts: hyperthyroidism, eye disease, and skin disease.

Most of the signs and symptoms of Graves' disease are the result of hyperthyroidism, which in turn results from the excessive production of thyroid hormones. Doctors can distinguish Graves' disease from other forms of hyperthyroidism because blood tests identify autoimmunity. In addition to the symptoms of hyperthyroidism detailed earlier in the chapter, autoimmunity can lead to eye disease and skin disease.

Causes of Graves' disease

In Chapter 5, I explain that about 10 percent of the world's population has thyroid autoantibodies, and these autoantibodies can lead to both hypothyroidism (underactive thyroid function) and hyperthyroidism. Some autoantibodies suppress the thyroid, and others stimulate it. If you have Graves' disease, the stimulating antibodies are in control in your body. Just why this happens is not clear, but doctors and researchers have a number of theories, including the following:

- The body makes many cells to prevent foreign tissue from invading and other cells that recognize the body's own tissue. When a patient has an autoimmune disorder, her body may have lost the cells meant to prevent other cells from reacting against the body's own tissue.

- Invading organisms such as viruses may share characteristics of normal body tissue. When the body creates antibodies to fight the invaders, those antibodies may react against normal tissue as well.

- Certain drugs can change the immunity of the body so it reacts against itself. The class of drugs that does this is called the *cytokines*. They are used in the treatment of hepatitis and leukemia, for example. Their effect is to activate or increase immunity. As a side effect, they may activate thyroid-stimulating immunity.

- Women, especially, may have genes that promote autoimmunity. The frequent occurrence of Graves' disease in mothers, daughters, and sisters confirms the genetic association (see Chapter 14).

- When the thyroid is injured, for example by a viral illness, it releases chemicals into the blood that are not normally found there. The protective immunity cells may make antibodies against those chemicals, which then react back at the thyroid.

- Iodine, given to a person with a large thyroid gland that was not making enough thyroid hormone previously (such as a multinodular goiter; see Chapter 9), can cause a sudden production of a lot of thyroid hormone that leads to hyperthyroidism.

- Stress can produce a rapid heart rate, sweating, and other signs similar to hyperthyroidism. Its role in the onset of hyperthyroidism is unclear.

Signs and symptoms specific to Graves' disease

Eye disease and skin disease associated with Graves' disease may be apparent even when a patient has no overt symptoms of hyperthyroidism. Sometimes eye and skin problems progress even after hyperthyroidism is under control. Severe forms of both these problems are rare, but thyroid eye disease can lead to blindness.

Thyroid eye disease

Thyroid eye disease, called *infiltrative ophthalmopathy* or *exopthalmus,* is present in almost all patients with Graves' disease. An ultrasound of the eye area can determine whether a patient has thyroid eye disease. Usually the condition is mild and does not progress after hyperthyroidism is controlled. Sometimes — in no more than 5 percent of Graves' patients — it does progress despite controlling the hyperthyroidism.

The patient with thyroid eye disease presents a clear-cut clinical picture. The eye, with its muscles and coverings, sits in a bony part of the skull called the *orbit.* When eye disease is present, the skin covering the eye and the muscles within the orbit are swelled and puffy. Since there is limited room within the orbit, the swollen skin and muscles are forced to push forward. Usually both eyes are affected, but the disease can start or progress more rapidly on one side than the other. If your eye is pushed forward far enough, your eyelids cannot close fully. The result is irritation and redness of the eyeball.

The optic nerve that carries the visual signal to your brain is stretched and sometimes damaged by thyroid eye disease, as is the back of the eye, the *retina,* where your eye focuses what it sees. The blood supply to these tissues can be compromised.

The eye muscles do not function properly, so that your eyes do not move together; you may experience double vision as a result. Occasionally, blindness may be the end result of all the damage.

When the eye muscles of a patient with thyroid eye disease are examined under a microscope, large numbers of autoimmune cells appear (similar to what is seen in the thyroid itself).

Treatment of thyroid eye disease is usually done in steps; severe measures are used only when milder measures fail. First, local measures like eye drops are given to treat the inflammation. If that fails to cure the problem, oral steroids are given to reduce your immunity. Other drugs that suppress immunity can be used.

Severe cases of thyroid eye disease usually respond to irradiation of the muscles in the orbit. If that does not work or the case is severe enough, a surgeon can remove bone from the orbit, thus decompressing the tissues.

While all this is going on, a doctor will attempt to remove all the patient's thyroid tissue so there will be no more antigens against which antibodies can be made, and the immune cells will decline. After the patient's thyroid is removed, she'll need to take thyroid hormone replacement pills. In theory, it would be helpful for the patient to take an antithyroid drug (which I describe later in the chapter) along with thyroid hormone replacement, because the antithyroid drugs decrease immunity, but this has not been carefully studied.

Thyroid skin disease

Thyroid skin disease, called *pretibial myxedema* and *thyroid acropachy,* is seen even less often than thyroid eye disease and is very severe in only 1 to 2 percent of patients with Graves' disease.

Pretibial myxedema is an abnormal thickening of the skin, usually in the front of the lower leg. Raised patches of skin are pink in appearance. The skin problems may last for several months or longer, then gradually improve. If they become severe, they may respond to steroids applied under tight dressings.

With *thyroid acropachy,* a patient's fingers become wider, and she may experience arthritic damage to the joints of the fingers. Fortunately, these lesions usually cause only unsightly fingers and no symptoms. Patients with these symptoms are not given any particular treatment.

Recognizing Other Causes of Hyperthyroidism

Although the vast majority of patients with hyperthyroidism have Graves' disease, about 20 percent do not. These patients may have one of several other conditions that lead to the increased production of free T4 and T3 (thyroid hormones). The treatment of these conditions may differ from treatment of Graves' disease, so it is important to recognize them.

Factitious (false) *hyperthyroidism* occurs when a patient is consuming large amounts of thyroid hormone without a doctor's knowledge. Usually some kind of psychological disturbance causes this behavior. The way to distinguish between this and other causes of hyperthyroidism is to check the size of the thyroid gland; a patient with factitious hyperthyroidism has a small thyroid gland. The gland is suppressed by the large amount of thyroid hormone. If a radioactive iodine uptake is done (see Chapter 4), this patient's thyroid gland won't absorb a great deal of the iodine.

A large thyroid with many nodules that is exposed to a lot of iodine may become hyperthyroid (see Chapter 9). Sometimes a single nodule may produce excessive amounts of thyroid hormone and cause the rest of the thyroid to shrink. These conditions can be felt by a doctor and confirmed by an ultrasound study or a thyroid scan (see Chapter 4).

Occasionally the thyroid produces large amounts of T3 but normal or even low levels of T4. This is a condition called *T3 thyrotoxicosis.* T3 thyrotoxicosis is an autoimmune condition and produces the same signs and symptoms and is treated in exactly the same way as Graves' disease (which is associated with a high free T4 level). This condition is really just Graves' disease with a predominance of T3. Doctors don't yet know why T3 is elevated in these cases rather than T4. If you have the signs and symptoms of hyperthyroidism but your free T4 level is normal or even low, your doctor should measure your T3 level.

A condition called *subacute thyroiditis* (see Chapter 11) may cause the release of a lot of thyroid hormone from the thyroid and briefly cause hyperthyroidism. The thyroid is usually tender, and the hyperthyroidism does not last.

Certain (not very common) tumors called *choriocarcinomas,* which arise from the placental tissue between a fetus and its mother, produce a lot of a hormone that stimulates the thyroid. This hormone, *human chorionic gonadotrophin,* can be measured in the blood.

Finally, central hyperthyroidism is also possible, although it occurs much less frequently than Graves' disease. Central hyperthyroidism is caused by too much thyrotrophin-releasing hormone from the hypothalamus in the brain or too much thyroid-stimulating hormone (TSH) from the pituitary gland in the brain (often as a result of a tumor). In this condition, the patient's TSH level is high (whereas with Graves' disease this level is low). The patient may experience symptoms of a brain tumor, such as headache or loss of part of the visual field.

Your doctor shouldn't have difficulty differentiating any of the conditions discussed in this section from Graves' disease, especially if he or she looks for signs that your eyes and skin are changing and orders tests that check for thyroid autoantibodies.

Choosing the Best Treatment for Graves' Disease

The treatment of Graves' disease has evolved over the years as doctors and researchers have come to understand it better and additional tools have become available. As soon as doctors understood that the thyroid was responsible for the excessive production of thyroid hormones, the obvious response was to cut out the offending tissue. This produced an era of great thyroid surgeons, along with a lot of unexpected problems that are described in the next section. Around 1950, surgery began to be replaced by the administration of radioactive iodine, which cured many patients but brought its own difficulties. Finally, antithyroid drugs became available.

Each form of treatment has its pros and cons. I find it interesting that doctors in Europe generally prefer antithyroid pills, while doctors in the U.S. choose radioactive iodine more often. In the following sections, I explain the advantages and disadvantages of each one, and I share with you my own bias regarding the best treatment options.

Thyroid surgery

Thyroid surgery involves the removal of part of the thyroid gland. Surgery quickly reduces the symptoms of hyperthyroidism by removing the source of those symptoms: the thyroid that was producing too much hormone.

With the availability of nonsurgical treatments, surgery is rarely done today for hyperthyroidism. Some situations leave surgery as the only choice, such as the following:

✔ The patient refuses to take radioactive iodine and develops an allergy or a bad reaction to antithyroid pills (or simply fails to take them).

✔ The thyroid gland is extremely large, which means that radioactive iodine or antithyroid pills may not be effective.

✔ Hyperthyroidism is diagnosed during pregnancy and cannot be controlled with antithyroid drugs, causing problems for the mother or the fetus. (Surgery can be done in the second trimester of the pregnancy.)

✔ The thyroid has nodules that suggest a possible cancer.

One reason why surgery is not often used to treat thyroid conditions these days is that surgery carries certain risks:

✔ Any surgical operation requiring anesthesia involves risk.

✔ Surgery can't be done on a person with severe heart or lung disease.

✔ Surgery can't be performed in the third trimester of pregnancy, because it could induce labor.

✔ Surgery can damage one or both *recurrent laryngeal nerves,* which can lead to hoarseness or permanent damage to the voice.

✔ Surgery can damage the *parathyroid glands* that lie behind the thyroid, leading to a severe drop in blood calcium.

✔ Although a surgeon's goal is to leave enough thyroid tissue to keep the patient's thyroid function normal, low thyroid function may begin immediately after surgery or develop during the next few years.

✔ If previous neck surgery has been done, it is risky to attempt another operation.

✔ The surgery is intricate, and a highly experienced surgeon is not always available.

Some specialists believe that surgery releases thyroid *antigens* (tissue or chemicals that the body is not normally exposed to) into the blood stream and leaves a lot of thyroid tissue intact, both of which can worsen the autoimmune condition, possibly resulting in worse eye disease. Whether or not this is true is unclear.

For more information about thyroid surgery, see Chapter 13.

Radioactive iodine treatment

In this treatment, a patient swallows a capsule containing radioactive iodine (RAI). Because the thyroid uses more iodine than any other organ or gland in the body, the RAI concentrates in the thyroid and slowly destroys the overactive thyroid cells.

It would seem that radioactive iodine is an ideal solution to the problem of hyperthyroidism. Decades of experience with radioactive iodine have lain to rest a number of the fears surrounding this treatment:

- ✔ There is no increase in thyroid cancer in adults who receive RAI.

- ✔ There is no increase in cases of leukemia after RAI.

- ✔ RAI does not affect reproductive ability.

- ✔ Children of mothers who previously received RAI have normal thyroid function and no congenital defects at birth (though RAI is never given during a pregnancy). These children can, however, still develop Graves' disease later in life because it is hereditary.

In addition, RAI is inexpensive and avoids the risks of surgery. But RAI does have its share of drawbacks:

- ✔ RAI can't be used for a pregnant woman because it crosses the placenta and enters the baby's thyroid, possibly destroying it.

- ✔ RAI should not be used in small children (younger than teenagers) because of the incidence of thyroid cancer when small children are exposed to it. (For example, thyroid cancer was rampant among children exposed to RAI outside the Russian nuclear plant at Chernobyl.)

- ✔ Finding the exact dose that will cure the hyperthyroidism but leave the patient with normal thyroid function is impossible. If too little RAI is used, another treatment is needed. Most patients given enough RAI to cure their hyperthyroidism will eventually become hypothyroid and need to take thyroid hormone replacement (possibly for life).

If RAI causes hypothyroidism, patients may experience three unusual symptoms: joint aches, stiffness, and headaches. The headaches may be due to swelling of the pituitary gland.

> ✔ By slowly destroying the thyroid, RAI releases a large amount of thyroid antigens into the patient's circulation, similar to what occurs in surgery, which may greatly increase autoimmunity and make eye disease worse.
>
> ✔ A patient must have follow-up blood tests for years to monitor for the development of hypothyroidism.

After RAI is given, it takes about three weeks to begin to have an effect, and it has its maximal effect about two months after treatment. (These timeframes can vary depending on how large the gland is when the treatment occurs.)

Antithyroid pills

There are two antithyroid pills used to control hyperthyroidism, *propylthiouricil* (PTU) and *methimazole*. Both pills block the production of thyroid hormones, but propylthiouricil also blocks the conversion of T4 to T3, giving it a theoretical advantage over methimazole. (This advantage does not seem to matter so much in practice unless you are trying to control the hyperthyroidism very rapidly.)

A major advantage of these pills is that, unlike surgery or radioactive iodine, they help to treat all complications of Graves' disease, including eye disease, by reducing autoimmunity. Also, given in correct dosages, they do not lead to hypothyroidism.

When either drug is given, the patient usually begins to feel better after three weeks, and the hyperthyroidism is controlled by six weeks. Then it is important to monitor the patient's free T4 level at least every six to eight weeks, because treatment can lower the T4 into the hypothyroid range.

Most patients are started on 5 milligrams of methimazole three times daily or 50 milligrams of propylthiouricil three times daily. As the patient's T4 level falls, the dose can be reduced to two pills or even one pill daily. The current standard is to keep the drug going for a year, and then to stop it to see whether the disease will recur.

At most, one-third of patients taking these pills will remain under control after they stop taking the propylthiouricil or methimazole. For the other two-thirds, the symptoms of hyperthyroidism recur after the pills are stopped. These patients can continue on antithyroid drugs or be treated by surgery or RAI.

Like surgery and RAI, these drugs carry some risks. The major risk is that they can cause a reduction in white blood cells and even, very rarely, a complete lack of white blood cell production (a condition called *agranulocytosis*). Although this usually occurs early in treatment when patients are given especially large doses of medication, it is occasionally seen later on and at low doses. This problem goes away when the patient stops taking the pill.

If you are on methimazole or propylthiouricil and develop a cold, sore throat, or other illness usually associated with a virus, contact your doctor, who should do a white blood cell count.

One way to avoid severe loss of white blood cell production is to have a white cell count done each time you visit your doctor while you are on these pills.

Another rare side effect of these drugs is the occurrence of liver function abnormalities and even liver damage. If you take one of these drugs, ask your doctor to check your liver function every few office visits.

Other helpful medications

Certain pills can reduce the symptoms of hyperthyroidism without treating the condition. They are valuable for controlling the disease while antithyroid pills or radioactive iodine has a chance to work. The major class of drugs is called *beta blockers,* and the most commonly used drug is *propranolol.* When given in a dose of 20 to 40 milligrams three to four times a day, it slows the heart, decreases anxiety, and reduces tremor. It can be continued for a few weeks until the other medications take effect, or it can be used as preparation for surgery.

My choice of treatment

For most patients with Graves' disease, methimazole is my first choice of treatment (or propylthiouricil for pregnant women). While it is true that only one-third of patients have a permanent remission after taking antithyroid drugs, the fact that the immune reaction is suppressed by these drugs (thus helping to reduce eye disease in hyperthyroidism) is an important reason for my choice. This is the only choice that may be truly curative and not simply destructive.

The largest thyroids I have seen have eventually responded to antithyroid drugs.

Many doctors cite the need to take a pill every day as a reason not to recommend antithyroid drugs. Most of these doctors give their patients radioactive iodine, and the patients often end up hypothyroid and needing to take daily thyroid hormone replacement pills, so I don't agree with this argument.

For other chronic illnesses such as diabetes or hypertension, patients take pills for a lifetime. I have never understood the reluctance to do the same thing with Graves' disease to avoid surgery and radioactive destruction of the thyroid gland. No rule says that pills cannot be given for more than a year. The pills also can be stopped on a yearly basis and not started again until the disease recurs, if it does.

If a patient is very symptomatic at the beginning of treatment, I use the beta blocker propranolol to control her symptoms until methimazole takes effect (in three to four weeks).

A patient who is stable on pills can be seen every few months, as long as she knows that she should contact the doctor if she experiences any symptoms of a virus, which may mean a reduction in her white blood cell count caused by the medication.

Preparations of iodine are used to temporarily block thyroid hormone production and reduce the blood flowing to the thyroid in preparation for surgery.

Treating Other Causes of Hyperthyroidism

Those people who have hyperthyroidism that is not caused by Graves' disease may need other treatment options:

- Factitious hyperthyroidism is treated by removing the thyroid pills from the patient and starting some form of psychotherapy.

- A thyroid with one or more nodules that produce too much thyroid hormone responds best to radioactive iodine, because the nodules are not caused by an autoimmune condition, so there is no concern about thyroid eye disease lingering after the treatment. In the case of a single nodule causing the hyperthyroidism, after the nodule is eliminated with RAI, the rest of the thyroid will often function normally. When single or multiple overactive nodules are present, antithyroid drugs almost never cause a permanent remission.

- T3 thyrotoxicosis responds to antithyroid medication just like Graves' disease caused by excess T4.

- The hyperthyroid phase of subacute thyroiditis does not last very long. If necessary, the beta blocker propranolol can control symptoms until the hyperthyroidism subsides.

- A choriocarcinoma making hormones that stimulate the thyroid must be removed.

- A tumor in the brain causing excessive production of thyroid-stimulating hormone must be treated by surgery or radiation therapy.

Surviving Thyroid Storm

Severe hyperthyroidism, known as *thyroid storm,* is a rare condition that may be fatal for the patient. The clinical picture is one of extreme signs and symptoms of hyperthyroidism. The patient has a high fever and very rapid heart beats. She may be vomiting, have diarrhea, and become dehydrated. She may be in heart failure and have a heart rhythm that cannot be controlled. She can be delirious and lapse into a coma.

Fortunately, this is rarely seen because hyperthyroidism is almost always diagnosed at a much earlier stage. It is sometimes seen when partially controlled hyperthyroidism is complicated by an infection. When it does occur, rapid treatment is essential.

This is a true medical emergency that should be managed by a physician who is very aware of the treatment of severe hyperthyroidism.

The doctor usually starts a number of treatments all at once. The patient is given fluids, one of the antithyroid drugs (such as propylthiouricil), potassium iodide, steroids, and a beta blocker like propranolol. This can lower the level of T3 hormone to normal in a day, although the patient takes many more days to fully recover.

If a patient does not respond to treatment, has a severe infection, or experiences a heart rhythm that cannot be controlled, this condition may be fatal.

Chapter 7

Thyroid Nodules

*I*n some ways the thyroid is really an annoying gland. If it were not so important to our health, there would be good reason to get rid of it, just like doctors used to get rid of tonsils. The thyroid is forever forming bumps and growths that turn out to be of little or no significance but have to be evaluated on the outside chance that they're cancerous. Even if a thyroid growth turns out to be cancerous (see Chapter 8), it's rarely fatal.

The reason we pay so much attention to the bumps on our thyroids is the same reason why a piece of property is valuable: location, location, location. If the thyroid gland weren't located so prominently in the front of the neck, all these little growths would never be noticed and most people would be no worse off for it. Instead, your thyroid got put right up front, thus providing a lifetime source of work and income for specialists who call themselves thyroidologists (like me).

This chapter tells you what you need to know about all these bumps and lumps. I explain whether you should be concerned or just ignore the nodule, as well as what to do if it becomes necessary to get rid of it. By the end of the chapter, I think you'll appreciate that most thyroid nodules are minor inconveniences, and knowing what to do about them will keep them that way.

What's a Thyroid Nodule?

Kenneth Fine is a 35-year-old man in excellent health. While shaving one day, he notices a bump on the front of his neck that he has not seen before. He ignores it for several months but finally decides that he ought to have someone check it out. He goes to his doctor, who does thyroid function tests. His free T4 and thyroid-stimulating hormone (TSH) levels are normal (see Chapter 4). His doctor then sends him to a thyroidologist for evaluation.

The thyroidologist asks Kenneth if the lump has grown noticeably and if it causes any trouble swallowing or breathing. Kenneth answers "no" to these questions. The specialist then proposes that Kenneth have a fine needle aspiration biopsy (see Chapter 4). When this test is done, the report comes back *benign thyroid adenoma,* which means that the lump is not cancerous. Kenneth is told to come back in a year for a reexamination.

A year later there has been no change, and the specialist asks him to return a year after that. Kenneth forgets about it and the doctor's receptionist has a poor bookkeeping system, so Kenneth lives happily ever after.

Kenneth is a very good example of the typical case history of a person with a thyroid nodule. He illustrates the unexpected finding of a bump, the tendency to ignore it, and the fact that it generally isn't a problem in the long run.

This case is not meant to minimize the fact that some nodules do turn out to be cancerous and must be dealt with in the proper way. This example simply illustrates the most common course of events.

The thyroid is ordinarily a smooth butterfly-shaped gland (see Chapter 3). Whenever something grows that alters that smoothness, the growth is considered a *nodule.*

Any new growth on the thyroid is called a *neoplasm.* Despite its harsh-sounding name, the term simply means "new growth." There may be one or several growths on a person's thyroid, and multiple explanations for why they appear. Physicians identify the various possibilities according to the appearance of the nodule tissue under a microscope. This is known as the *pathological appearance* of the tissue. For our purposes, we just want to know whether the nodule is *benign* (not cancerous) or *malignant* (cancerous).

Most thyroid nodules — *more than 90 percent* — are benign.

Evaluating Cancer Risks

A number of facts about a patient's history, signs, and symptoms can help sway the balance towards or away from a diagnosis of cancer:

- If a patient has many nodules, this suggests that a cancer is not present. Most multinodular thyroids are found to be benign.

- A most important point in a patient's history is previous exposure to irradiation. (This does not include the use of radioactive iodine in the treatment of hyperthyroidism — see Chapter 6.) A significant increase in thyroid cancer has been reported in children exposed to the radiation from the Chernobyl Nuclear Plant in Russia. In this case, multiple nodules do not rule out cancer. Almost half the nodules in an irradiated gland turn out to be cancer.

✔ A nodule that grows rapidly is probably a cancer, but if it pops up suddenly and is tender, it may be a hemorrhage. A hemorrhage like this is not usually a serious problem, but it does cause discomfort.

✔ Nodules are found less often in men than women but are cancerous more often in men, when they are found.

✔ Nodules found in children are cancerous more frequently than they are in adults. However, a nodule in a child is still benign more often than it is malignant.

✔ There is virtually no family or hereditary connection with nodules, either benign or cancerous. The exception is a condition called *multiple endocrine neoplasia* where many members of a family have nodules on several different glands such as the thyroid, the pancreas, the parathyroids, and the adrenal glands.

✔ Symptoms of hoarseness and trouble swallowing suggest cancer.

✔ Finding growths in the neck away from the thyroid suggests cancer that has spread, and those growths must be evaluated by a biopsy.

✔ If the thyroid does not move freely, it is a sign of fixation that suggests cancer.

Securing a Diagnosis

If the questions in the previous section don't provide enough evidence suggesting whether a nodule is cancerous or not, your doctor can use several tests to make a diagnosis.

Thyroid function tests

Thyroid function tests that suggest hyperthyroidism (see Chapter 6) or hypothyroidism (see Chapter 5) usually mean that a thyroid nodule is benign. However, the possibility exists for two different conditions to be present in the thyroid at the same time. Therefore, your doctor should examine the nodule occasionally to guarantee that it is not growing.

The thyroid scan

A thyroid scan (see Chapter 4) can distinguish a nodule that takes up radioactive iodine from one that does not. A nodule may be actively concentrating the iodine even though the thyroid function tests are normal. A "warm" nodule takes up radioactive iodine like the rest of the gland. If the nodule concentrates most of the iodine (while the rest of the gland is less active) and the thyroid function tests are elevated, it is a "hot" nodule. Cancerous nodules are usually "cold," meaning they do not concentrate the radioactivity. However, most cold nodules are not cancerous.

Figure 7-1 shows the typical appearance of a cold nodule and a hot nodule.

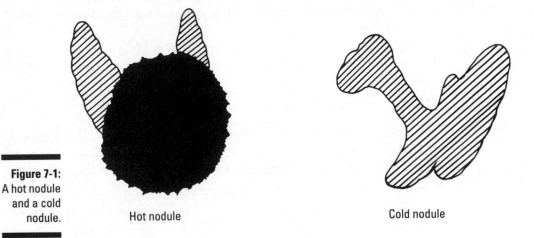

Figure 7-1:
A hot nodule and a cold nodule.

Hot nodule   Cold nodule

In addition, the thyroid scan will sometimes show multiple nodules when only one was seen or felt. Multiple nodules argue against a cancer.

The thyroid ultrasound study

The *thyroid ultrasound study* (see Chapter 4) also gives a picture of the entire thyroid and demonstrates if more than one nodule is present. More helpful than that, the ultrasound can distinguish between a solid mass and a cyst. A cyst is a nodule that is either filled with fluid or contains some solid tissue. A cyst filled with fluid is generally believed to be a benign growth. A cyst that contains some solid tissue may be a cancer.

The fine needle aspiration biopsy

This test is the gold standard for the diagnosis of a thyroid nodule. Often specialists will skip the other steps and go right to this simple, painless, and very specific procedure. A tiny needle is stuck into the nodule, and bits of tissue are removed from it. Doctors believe that this test gives the correct diagnosis 98 percent of the time.

Thyroid cancers tend to grow either very slowly or so fast that they are obvious. If they grow fast, the biopsy is done immediately. If they grow slowly, the fine needle aspiration biopsy can be done a year or more after a slowly growing nodule is discovered, still leaving plenty of time to treat a newly discovered cancer. Of course, the doctor must check for evidence of changes in the key findings discussed earlier in the chapter each time the patient is seen, such as the development of hoarseness, the finding of a new growth away from the thyroid in the neck, or fixation of a thyroid that previously moved freely.

Treating Cancerous Nodules

Every so often one of these anonymous nodules turns out to be a cancer (see Chapter 8), and treatment becomes necessary. (Sometimes all the tests available to a doctor do not provide a definitive diagnosis, in which case I believe it's wise to treat the nodule as if it were cancer.)

The treatment of choice for a cancerous thyroid nodule is surgery. Even benign nodules may sometimes require surgery if they are unsightly or cause compression or trouble with swallowing.

When a doctor and patient determine that surgery is necessary, two key requirements must be met:

✔ A competent surgeon with plenty of experience in thyroid surgery must be available. The potential complications of thyroid surgery are discussed in Chapter 13. No general surgeon who does only occasional thyroid cases should undertake thyroid surgery for potential cancer, because the cancer may be very extensive. Furthermore, the right procedure must be done the first time around, because a second surgery would be much more difficult and complicated.

If you need to have thyroid surgery, check the qualifications of the surgeon. Do not accept a referral without checking the surgeon's experience and rate of complications.

✔ There must be a competent and experienced pathologist at the hospital where surgery is to be performed. The reason for this is that the pathologist will be called upon to give a diagnosis of the tissue that the surgeon removes as surgery proceeds. The pathologist's opinion determines whether the surgeon will do a complete removal of the thyroid (called a *total thyroidectomy*) and will then go on to remove lymph nodes in the neck around the thyroid to see if the cancer has spread. This extensive (and expensive) operation should not be done unless the pathologist can give the surgeon a precise diagnosis. Ideally, the final diagnosis of the tissue, made after surgery is complete, will not contradict the diagnosis made during the operation.

You probably will not find highly experienced pathologists at community hospitals, even though many thyroid cancers are discovered at these hospitals. Do yourself or your loved one a major favor and go to a referral center to get this special care.

A few thyroid specialists would argue that even if a nodule is diagnosed as cancerous, the patient is better off if the nodule is left alone. They base this argument on the fact that although about 15,000 new cases of thyroid cancer are detected in the United States each year, only 1,500 people in the U.S. die from thyroid cancer each year. Furthermore, the 15,000 new cases of thyroid cancer are derived from as many as 15 million people with nodules of one kind or another. Because death from thyroid cancer is such a rare event, some specialists reason that treatment may not matter. Most evidence does not support this.

I believe that nodules that contain thyroid cancer should be treated, but I keep an open mind because I know people who have opinions that differ.

Dealing with Nodules That Are Not Cancer

Hot nodules and benign cysts may require some treatment, but not necessarily surgery. It is almost always preferable to deal with the thyroid nonsurgically if the results will be satisfactory because of the potential for surgical complications, not to mention the cost and the trauma that surgery brings with it. Fortunately, other treatment choices are available for nodules that are not cancerous, and new ones are being discovered regularly.

Hot nodules

A hot nodule produces hyperthyroidism, so it must be treated. One choice is to give the patient radioactive iodine (RAI), as is done for Graves' disease (see Chapter 6). However, up to 40 percent of the patients treated with RAI develop hypothyroidism (underactive thyroid) later in life. Those who do not develop hypothyroidism will usually return to normal thyroid function.

A newer treatment that eliminates the hot nodule while not destroying the rest of the thyroid gland is the injection of ethanol into the nodule. This is done several times over several days. Complications include pain in the thyroid area and fever. This treatment may be used more and more often in the future as doctors gain experience with it.

Benign cysts

A nodule that is filled with fluid will shrink when a needle is inserted and the fluid is removed. Unfortunately, the cyst often fills right up again. Repeated removal of the fluid sometimes cures the problem. Ethanol can be injected into a cyst just as it can be injected into a solid nodule. The cyst may also be left alone if you are willing to live with it.

Warm or cold nodules

Nodules that do not produce excessive thyroid hormone and are not cancer are sometimes treated by giving thyroid hormone to the patient in an attempt to shrink the nodule. Little evidence has been found that this treatment actually works. Very rarely have I found these nodules to respond to thyroid hormone. The risk involved is that giving too much thyroid hormone could cause bone loss or abnormal heart beats.

Sometimes, when even a fine needle biopsy does not produce a definite diagnosis, the doctor suggests using thyroid hormone suppression. If a patient consumes thyroid hormone and the nodule shrinks, then the doctor assumes that the nodule is not a cancer. If the nodule does not shrink, the suspicion of a cancer is greater. I disagree with this method, because most nodules do not respond to thyroid hormone, yet most nodules are not cancer.

Warm and cold nodules should be examined every six months or every year. Should the nodule grow, a fine needle biopsy is done again. Otherwise, it can be left alone.

Ignoring Small Nodules

Every so often a study, such as an ultrasound of the neck, reveals one or more very small nodules on the thyroid. The best specialists probably cannot feel a nodule that is less than one centimeter in size. The ultrasound may detect a half-centimeter or smaller nodule. My advice is to ignore a bump this small, which has been termed an *incidentaloma* (a thyroid specialist's agonizing attempt at humor).

Chapter 8

Thyroid Cancer

- -

- -

For me, this chapter is probably the hardest one to write. The word *cancer* evokes a number of images, and none of them are particularly positive. The fact is that people do die of thyroid cancer. For this reason, you must know what thyroid cancer is, how it grows, how you treat it, and how you follow up after treatment if you or a loved one has thyroid cancer. But it's also important to put thyroid cancer into perspective.

Researchers estimate that as much as 6 percent of the world's population has cancer in the thyroid gland. Based on this percentage, about 16.5 million people in the United States may have evidence of thyroid cancer. Yet in the U.S., only 15,000 new cases are found each year, and the total deaths due to thyroid cancer each year are 1,500 to 2,000. The vast majority of people with thyroid cancer live and die without ever knowing that it exists. The cancer is detected only when the thyroid is carefully examined under a microscope.

Thyroid cancer does not appear among the top 75 causes of death in the United States. Among cancers, thyroid cancer is not in the top 15 causes of death. This suggests that compared to most other cancers, thyroid cancer is one of the least dangerous. If you had to have a cancer, this might be the one to choose.

The relatively benign course of most thyroid cancer makes it difficult to say which treatment is best. Perhaps certain treatments are very effective, or perhaps any number of treatments would work just as well because the disease itself is so mild. For this reason, there is much difference of opinion among thyroid specialists. If you ask two thyroid specialists how to treat a certain type of thyroid cancer, you may get three opinions of what to do. In this chapter, I give you my recommendations based upon the best and most recent investigations of thyroid cancer treatment.

Determining What Causes Thyroid Cancer

John D'Mee is 40 years of age and has noticed that he has a lump in the front of his neck on the left side. His family has no history of thyroid cancer. The lump is painless and moves when he swallows. He does not know how long it has been there. John goes to see his doctor, who does thyroid function tests and finds that the TSH and free T4 are normal. He does a thyroid scan and finds that the area of the nodule on John's thyroid does not take up any radioactivity — it's a *cold* nodule. John's doctor sends him to see Dr. Rubin, who does a fine needle aspiration biopsy (see Chapter 4). The pathologist diagnoses a *papillary carcinoma*, the most common type of thyroid cancer. Dr. Rubin sends John to a head and neck surgeon who has done more than 2,000 thyroid surgeries.

The surgeon, Dr. Stark, recommends removing the thyroid gland while carefully retaining the tissue around the parathyroid glands and the recurrent laryngeal nerves that pass along the thyroid. The surgery is done, successfully, and no other suspicious nodes or nodules are found during the procedure.

John has no other treatment initially. He returns to Dr. Rubin, and three weeks after surgery, he has a TSH test. The result is very high — 45 — indicating that there's little thyroid tissue remaining in his body. He has another scan that shows no uptake of radioactive iodine except for in a small area of the thyroid tissue that was left intact by the surgeon. John is given a large dose of radioactive iodine to eliminate that small bit of tissue. A follow-up scan shows that all the thyroid tissue is gone. John is placed on thyroid hormone replacement and continues to be monitored by Dr. Rubin. John will probably live a normal life span with no further trouble associated with the thyroid cancer other than the periodic visits for follow-up.

John is representative of the majority of people who develop thyroid cancer. The cancer shows itself as a thyroid nodule (see Chapter 7). Keep in mind that the vast majority of thyroid nodules are *not* cancerous.

Our understanding of why cancer occurs is becoming clearer and clearer. We know that genes (part of our hereditary makeup) called *oncogenes* cause a cell to grow and divide without controls. Oncogenes exist in all of our cells. Just exactly what permits certain oncogenes to begin to be active is not clear, but it could be a mistake in cell division (a *mutation*), or it could be some chemical or radiation in the environment.

Other genes called *tumor suppressor genes* have been found in the human chromosome (the *DNA*). Some people lack these tumor suppressor genes and can develop tumors.

The best-known initiator of thyroid cancer is irradiation, which has been the source of many cancers in children who lived in the area of Chernobyl in Russia. The children drank milk from cows that ate the grass upon which radioactive substances (including radioactive iodine) fell. Within a few years, many of the children had multiple sites of cancer in their thyroid glands. Adults exposed to radioactive iodine also developed thyroid cancer, though not as often as children, who seem to be more sensitive.

Children who have received neck and face irradiation for benign conditions such as acne or enlarged tonsils have also developed thyroid cancer. In this case, the cancer occurs as many as 40 years later.

Some cancers of the thyroid run in families, especially the cancer called *medullary thyroid cancer*. I discuss this hereditary connection later in the chapter.

Identifying the Types of Thyroid Cancer

A pathologist identifies thyroid cancer according to the appearance of the tissue that he or she examines. If a nodule is diagnosed as cancer, it's important to identify the particular cancer, since each one follows a different course. Treatments that work for one type of thyroid cancer may not work at all for a different type.

As a patient, you do not need to know how to identify these types of cancer — that's the pathologist's job. But a basic understanding of the types of cancer will help you know what the future holds if a thyroid cancer is identified. When your doctor tells you the name of the cancer, you will have an idea of what to expect.

The descriptions for each type of thyroid cancer are true for most patients with that type of cancer, but there are exceptions. Once in a while, people with the most aggressive type of thyroid cancer will find that their cancer is not as aggressive as expected. By the same token, once in a while, a more benign form of thyroid cancer (based upon its appearance) will take a more aggressive turn. Medicine is not an exact science.

Papillary thyroid cancer

Papillary thyroid cancer is the most common form that thyroid cancer takes, accounting for more than 70 percent of thyroid cancers in both adults and children. Fortunately, this form of thyroid cancer also tends to take a benign course, meaning it's not very aggressive. Although it spreads to the local lymph glands in the neck as often as half the time, the spread does not seem to make the cancer more aggressive.

How a pathologist identifies a cancer

The pathologist looks for a number of abnormalities that separate normal tissue from cancerous tissue. He or she has studied thousands of tissue slides and knows the appearance of the tissue when it's found in a person whose clinical course suggests cancer compared with a person who has a benign clinical course. The key things that the pathologist looks for are:

✔ A malignant appearance to the tissue, which means very large, abnormal looking cells containing abnormal looking parts.

✔ The presence of even normal looking tissue in an area where it does not belong, which suggests that it has invaded that area. Examples are thyroid cells in a lymph gland, in bone, or in the lung.

The most important characteristics of papillary thyroid cancer are:

✔ It rarely spreads away from the neck.

✔ It's diagnosed most commonly between the ages of 30 and 50.

✔ Females have papillary cancer three times as often as males.

✔ It's the thyroid cancer most often associated with radiation exposure.

✔ It concentrates radioactive iodine, which can be used to destroy it.

✔ Patients over age 45 may have a more aggressive course, especially if the tumor is larger than 1 centimeter.

✔ It's especially mild in younger patients, very rarely causing death.

Follicular thyroid cancer

Follicular thyroid cancer makes up another 20 percent of all thyroid cancers. It's a little more aggressive than papillary cancer, but still usually takes a benign course. It does not tend to spread locally to lymph glands, but goes to bone and the lungs more often than papillary cancer. Its central features are:

✔ It's diagnosed most often between the ages of 40 and 60.

✔ Females are affected three times as often as males.

✔ It concentrates radioactive iodine.

✔ It invades blood vessels, accounting for its tendency to go to distant sites.

✔ It tends to be more aggressive in older patients.

There's another cancer that follows a course similar to follicular cancer but has a different appearance under the microscope. It's called a *Hurthle cell tumor.* It does not tend to concentrate radioactive iodine, so this cannot be used in treatment.

Medullary thyroid cancer

Medullary thyroid cancer makes up only about 5 percent of all cancers of the thyroid gland.

This cancer does not arise in the cells that produce thyroid hormones; rather, it arises in another type of cell found in the thyroid, called the *C cell.* The C cell produces a chemical (a hormone) called *calcitonin,* which does not affect metabolism. This is useful because, after this cancer is treated by completely removing the thyroid, the calcitonin level can be measured. If calcitonin levels are measured at regular intervals, a recurrence of cancer can be diagnosed easily.

Medullary thyroid cancer differs from the others in its occasional tendency to run in families. Eighty percent of the time no other family member has it. Twenty percent of the time it's found in a hereditary form. Either another member of the family will also have medullary thyroid cancer or the patient herself or himself will have the medullary thyroid cancer as part of a condition called *Multiple Endocrine Neoplasia* (MEN) *Syndrome.*

Two different types of MEN exist. Patients with MEN type II-A have tumors of the adrenal medulla (called *pheochromocytoma*) and the parathyroid glands in the neck. The adrenal medulla makes a hormone called *epinephrine,* so these patients get high blood pressure. They also get elevated levels of calcium as a result of the parathyroid tumor. MEN type II-B also includes the adrenal tumor that produces excessive amounts of epinephrine but not the parathyroid tumor. The third feature of MEN II-B is a characteristic physical appearance with tumors in the mouth.

If your diagnosis is medullary cancer of the thyroid, a doctor must check to see if you have tumors in the adrenal medulla, because such tumors must be controlled with medication before surgery. Otherwise your blood pressure could be high, making surgery on your neck extremely dangerous.

The important characteristics of medullary thyroid cancer include:

- ✔ It's found in women more often than in men.
- ✔ It's not associated with exposure to radiation.
- ✔ It's more aggressive than papillary or follicular thyroid cancers, especially if it spreads to the lymph glands in the neck or to the bone and liver.

✔ If one family member is diagnosed with medullary thyroid cancer, other family members should have their calcitonin levels checked. If a family member's calcitonin is elevated, he or she should have the thyroid removed because cancer is almost always found or, if not yet present, will develop later.

✔ Even when the calcitonin is not elevated in a family member, genetic testing can determine whether that person may eventually get a medullary thyroid cancer (see Chapter 14).

✔ Measuring calcitonin levels reveals whether a tumor has spread or recurred after the removal of the thyroid.

Some thyroid specialists advocate measuring calcitonin as a screening test for all nodules suspected to contain thyroid cancer. So far, this is not being done.

After 10 years, about 50 percent of patients with medullary thyroid cancer who receive treatment are still alive.

Undifferentiated (anaplastic) cancer

Fortunately, *undifferentiated cancer* is very rare, accounting for only about 2 percent of all thyroid cancers. This type of cancer is very aggressive and rarely cured. While 95 percent or more of patients with papillary or follicular thyroid cancer will be alive and doing well after 10 years, less than 10 percent of patients with undifferentiated thyroid cancer will be alive after three years.

This cancer is aggressive and invasive. While lymph node invasion by papillary cancer is not a bad sign, lymph node invasion by undifferentiated cancer predicts a bad outcome.

The cancer tends to attach to local structures like the nearby muscles, the trachea, the esophagus, and the blood vessels, making surgery very difficult, if not impossible. The outlook is so bad that there's little justification for extensive surgery that just mutilates the patient without accomplishing a cure.

Important features of this cancer include:

✔ Males are afflicted twice as often as females.

✔ It usually occurs in patients over the age of 65.

✔ It may occur in patients with a distant history of radiation to the neck or face.

✔ By the time it's diagnosed, it has already spread to local nodes and distant structures like the lungs, bone, brain, and liver.

✔ Most people will die of this cancer within six months or a year of diagnosis.

The Stages of Thyroid Cancer

For purposes of treatment, thyroid cancers are *staged* (divided into stages). This means that they are divided up by whether the cancer remains within the thyroid, whether and where spread has taken place, and whether the tumor moves or is attached to surrounding tissues. It's important to know which stage a cancer is in, because a follicular cancer that has the same stage as a papillary cancer responds to treatment in the same way, while two follicular cancers at very different stages respond differently:

- ✔ **Stage I:** The tumor is entirely within the thyroid gland with no spread to other areas.

- ✔ **Stage II:** A tumor is in the thyroid but also has spread to the local lymph nodes. Both the thyroid and the lymph nodes are freely movable. The tumor has not become attached to surrounding tissues.

- ✔ **Stage III:** The tumor and/or lymph nodes are attached to the surrounding tissues.

- ✔ **Stage IV:** The tumor has spread outside the neck.

Treating the Stages of Thyroid Cancer

Most treatment of thyroid cancer initially involves surgery. The experience and competence of the surgeon is extremely important, no matter what stage of cancer the patient has.

The most controversial treatment involves stage I thyroid cancer, because it's hard to know if the treatment itself or the benign course of the disease is responsible for a good outcome. General agreement exists about the best way to treat the other stages, but even there some disagreement exists. In the following sections, I try to offer the most generally accepted treatment recommendations, but of course anyone facing treatment must talk with an internist and surgeon to get their perspective.

Stage 1

Because the size of the tumor plays a role in the prognosis, different levels of surgery are recommended depending upon whether the tumor is less than or greater than 1 centimeter in size.

The smaller tumor is treated by removing the lobe of the thyroid in which it's found, plus partially removing the other lobe, leaving some tissue intact (including the tissue that is next to the parathyroid glands and the recurrent laryngeal nerve). The larger tumor is usually treated by removing the entire thyroid, with the exception of the tissue adjacent to the parathyroid glands and recurrent laryngeal nerve. Both operations are intended to ensure that the patient's parathyroid glands will continue to function and that his or her speech will not be damaged after surgery. The difference between the two is that the first operation leaves part of the thyroid intact because the chance that the cancer has spread to the other lobe is small.

Some thyroid specialists recommend the smaller operation for any stage I thyroid tumor, regardless of size. This is because of the generally good prognosis of any stage I tumor. It has not been proved that more surgery is better in this case.

If even a small tumor has developed as a result of receiving radiation to the thyroid, the patient should have the larger operation (removal of the entire thyroid) because usually cancer can be found in both lobes.

A patient who has most of his or her thyroid removed (the larger operation) is kept off thyroid hormone treatment. If any thyroid cancer remains, a radioactive iodine scan detects it, and it can be treated with a large dose of radioactive iodine. This destroys all remaining thyroid tissue, which can be proved by a subsequent scan, and makes it easier to diagnose and treat a recurrence of the thyroid cancer in the future.

Stage II

Thyroidologists generally agree about the correct treatment for stage II thyroid cancer: An experienced surgeon should remove as much of the thyroid as possible, preserving the parathyroid glands and the recurrent laryngeal nerves. The surgeon also looks for enlarged nodes in the neck, which are removed. If cancer is found in these nodes, the surgeon removes as many of the nodes in the local area of the neck as he or she can find.

After surgery, the patient is kept off thyroid hormone treatment for three weeks, and then the level of TSH is measured. If it's above 20, a thyroid scan is done to look for any residual thyroid tissue. Any tissue found is removed by giving a large dose of radioactive iodine. The patient is then placed on enough thyroid hormone to keep the TSH at the bottom of the normal range (around 0.3). This is done because it's believed that even thyroid cancer responds to TSH stimulation, and the object is to prevent further growth of the cancer.

Stage III

Since the tumor has invaded the local structures, more extensive surgery is needed to treat stage III thyroid cancer. The need for a highly experienced surgeon is even greater in this situation. There may be invasion of the tumor into the wall of the *trachea* (windpipe), and part of this must be removed. If there's tumor in muscle, this is removed. As much of the tumor as possible must be removed without disfiguring the patient. Because the cells of this tumor are so abnormal, they often do not take up radioactive iodine, so this form of treatment cannot be used. Instead, external irradiation is often given if much tumor has to be left in the neck during the surgery.

Stage IV

If possible, the surgeon removes any distinct areas where the tumor has spread away from the thyroid outside the neck. In addition, the thyroid is completely removed, as are the lymph glands in the neck. If the spread of cancer is very wide, an attempt is made to get the distant tumor to take up radioactive iodine after the thyroid is removed. If the tumor does not take up radioactive iodine, it's treated with external irradiation.

Medullary thyroid cancer

This type of cancer isn't a tumor that originates in thyroid-producing cells, so its treatment is a little different. A surgeon removes the entire thyroid, because the fact that medullary carcinoma does not concentrate iodine means radioactive iodine cannot be used to eliminate thyroid tissue. The surgeon also removes lymph nodes in the neck that contain tumor. External irradiation may be used in this situation. The patient's calcitonin level is measured at intervals to check for any regrowth of tumor.

Family members of a patient with medullary carcinoma should have their calcitonin levels checked, and if their levels are high, they should seek treatment as well. Genetic testing can also be done to rule out medullary thyroid cancer in other family members.

Following Up Cancer Treatment

Any patient who has most or all of her thyroid removed must start taking a thyroid hormone replacement after the surgery and will need to continue that treatment for the rest of her life. As I discuss in Chapter 5, thyroid hormone replacement simply involves taking a daily pill.

Patients who are treated for stage I or II thyroid cancer should have their blood levels of thyroglobulin (see Chapter 3) checked regularly after surgery. If the level starts to rise, thyroid hormone replacement is stopped for several weeks. A full body scan with radioactive iodine is done, looking for any evidence of thyroid tissue. If tissue is found, the patient is given a much larger treatment dose of radioactive iodine, which destroys the remaining thyroid tissue. The replacement thyroid hormone is restarted a few days later.

Stopping the thyroid hormone allows the body to produce thyroid-stimulating hormone (TSH), which stimulates uptake of radioactive iodine by thyroid tissue. Instead of stopping thyroid hormone replacement, your doctor could give you synthetic TSH injections for several days prior to a thyroid scan with almost as good a result.

Patients with stage III or IV thyroid cancer will probably show regrowth of tumor. This may respond to more external irradiation or to chemicals known to kill the tumor. The outlook is poor for patients who have recurrent stage III or IV thyroid cancer.

Chapter 9

Multinodular Goiters: Thyroids with Many Nodules

In This Chapter

▶ Knowing what causes a multinodular goiter

▶ Diagnosing and treating the problem

▶ Dealing with unexpected complications

Multinodular goiters — large thyroids with many nodules — may well be the most common of all thyroid disorders. In various studies of thyroid glands of people who died of other causes, between 30 and 60 percent of the glands have been found to have multiple nodules. That means as many as 165 million people in the United States alone have this disorder. What a bonanza for thyroid specialists! (With numbers like that, you have to wonder whose idea it was to place the thyroid gland so prominently in the front of the neck near so many vital structures and to make it so important. I would call it bad planning.)

Fortunately (or unfortunately, depending on which side of the desk you are sitting on), most of these people will never be seen or treated for their thyroid nodules. Only a small fraction will develop the signs and symptoms discussed in this chapter and need to be evaluated.

A Multinodular Goiter Grows Up

Ryan Fine (a distant cousin of our friend Kenneth from Chapter 7) is 46 years old. He goes to his doctor for a routine physical examination, and the doctor tells him that his thyroid feels bumpy. He has no symptoms in his neck. His doctor obtains thyroid function tests, which are normal, and thyroid autoantibody tests, which are negative. He is referred to the specialist, the venerable Dr. Rubin.

Dr. Rubin examines Ryan and tells him that he can feel several distinct nodules, all of them soft and freely moveable. He sends Ryan for a thyroid scan, which shows that all the nodules can concentrate radioactive iodine (none of them are "cold" — see Chapter 7). Dr. Rubin assures Ryan that he has a multinodular goiter and that no treatment is needed as long as he is free of symptoms. He asks Ryan to return in six months so that he can examine the thyroid again.

Four months later, Ryan suddenly feels pain in his neck and notices that one area has gotten larger. He goes to see Dr. Rubin, who inserts a needle in that area and removes a small amount of blood. He tells Ryan that a hemorrhage has occurred in one of the nodules, forming a cyst (a fluid-filled nodule) that requires no more treatment than evacuation of the blood. This happens once more, and then it stops. Ryan returns every six months thereafter, and there is no further change.

Ryan is an excellent illustration of the way that a multinodular goiter is typically discovered and evaluated and the most common outcome of the condition. Doctors believe that multinodular goiters result from some or all of the following circumstances:

- Starting around puberty, sometimes related to a deficiency of iodine (see Chapter 12), the thyroid is stimulated to grow. It grows a certain amount and then enters a resting state. This growth/resting cycle is repeated many times.

- The cells in the thyroid, though they almost all perform the same task of making thyroid hormone, are not identical and grow at different rates.

- Certain stresses to the body, such as a pregnancy, increase the need for iodine, leading to more stimulation of the thyroid.

- Some foods called *goitrogens* (see Chapter 5) prevent the production of thyroid hormone and lead to more stimulation of the thyroid.

- Certain drugs, such as amiodarone (taken for heart rhythm irregularities), block production of thyroid hormone, which leads to more growth of the thyroid to compensate.

- There may be a genetic connection so that multinodular goiters occur more often in some families than in others.

Figure 9-1 shows what a multinodular goiter looks like in comparison to a normal thyroid.

Ryan illustrates one way in which the goiter is discovered, but goiters may be found in many ways, including the following:

- A large neck suddenly gets much larger, leading to a visit to the doctor.

- Someone feels a sudden pain in his neck, and one side of his neck becomes larger because there is bleeding in a nodule.

✔ A doctor feels a large thyroid with many nodules during a routine examination.

✔ Symptoms develop such as a cough, difficulty swallowing, a feeling of pressure in the neck, or a lump in the throat.

✔ The goiter is discovered incidentally when other testing is done like an ultrasound study of the neck or an X-ray of the chest.

✔ Occasionally, particularly in older people, the patient has a heart irregularity or signs and symptoms of hyperthyroidism (see Chapter 6).

Figure 9-1:
A multinodular goiter compared to a normal thyroid.

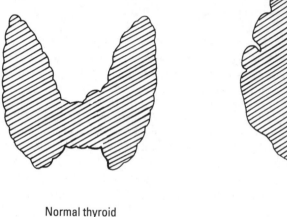
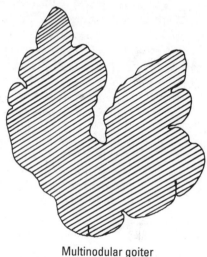

Normal thyroid   Multinodular goiter

Choosing to Treat It or Ignore It

Multinodular goiters generally proceed along the same path in most patients. When thyroid function tests are done, the results are either normal or the thyroid hormone levels are possibly elevated, suggesting hyperthyroidism; the thyroid hormone levels are rarely low. If a patient experiences sudden pain in one area of the thyroid, the doctor performs a *fine needle aspiration biopsy* (see Chapter 4). Usually that area of the thyroid contains blood as a result of a hemorrhage in one of the nodules. When the blood is removed, the nodule shrinks.

If a particular nodule stands out or is harder than the others, it is biopsied and usually found to be benign. If the nodule is cancerous, treatment for cancer is begun (see Chapter 8).

If the only problem is the large gland, most of the time the doctor doesn't treat it. If the patient experiences other symptoms in the neck or if the thyroid gland is particularly unsightly, the doctor treats the gland.

Sometimes the thyroid, instead of growing up and out, grows downward behind the chest bone (the *sternum*) and is said to be *substernal*. In this position, where there is little room to grow, it can squeeze other organs like the *trachea*, the air pipe from the nose to the lungs. Treatment may be necessary to reduce symptoms that arise from this condition.

Most people with a multinodular goiter don't realize they have it, and even if they're aware that it exists, they don't find treating it necessary.

Making a Diagnosis

Depending upon how a multinodular goiter is discovered, a doctor can do a number of studies to determine exactly what is going on in the thyroid gland.

A good pair of expert hands can feel the presence of many nodules (although no one can feel nodules smaller than a centimeter in size). This examination is very important because it serves as a baseline for future thyroid exams. The doctor notes the size of the thyroid so he can compare what he feels during future examinations to determine if the thyroid is growing.

The first study of a multinodular goiter consists of thyroid function tests to see whether enough thyroid hormone is being made. These test results are usually normal, but occasionally they show excess production of thyroid hormone. Thyroid autoantibody tests are sometimes done, especially if the patient has a family history of goiter. These test results are usually negative unless autoimmune thyroiditis is present (see Chapter 5).

If thyroid function tests indicate hyperthyroidism, the doctor looks for other signs of hyperthyroidism due to Graves' disease. Thyroid eye and skin disease, described in Chapter 6, would support a diagnosis of Graves' disease. A patient who has hyperthyroidism in a multinodular goiter has a condition called *toxic multinodular goiter,* also known as *Plummer's disease.*

When one nodule stands out or is harder than the others, the doctor does a fine needle aspiration biopsy to rule out cancer. A thyroid scan may precede the biopsy to see whether the nodule is functional (warm or hot) or if it is cold (see Chapter 7). Cancers are usually cold. However, keep in mind that the majority of cold nodules are not cancer. If cancer isn't present, the fine needle biopsy doesn't add any information that points to a diagnosis of the multinodular goiter.

A thyroid scan gives a general picture of the thyroid, showing the size of the gland, the many nodules, and the position of the gland, which is particularly important if it is below the sternum (as I explain in the previous section).

A thyroid ultrasound picks up very small nodules. This test can be used to show whether a tender nodule is a cyst — a fluid-filled nodule.

If a patient feels significant pressure in his neck or has trouble swallowing, the doctor may order a *barium swallow:* The patient swallows barium, and X-rays are taken as it passes down. This test may show that the thyroid gland is putting pressure on the *esophagus,* the swallowing tube from the mouth to the stomach. A plain film (without barium) of the neck reveals if the trachea is deviated by the mass of the thyroid.

Thyroid function tests should always be done when a patient has a multinodular goiter. Depending upon the stress the patient feels from this growth in the neck and upon how important the doctor thinks it is to leave no stone unturned, many, all, or none of the other tests described in this section may be done.

Treating a Multinodular Goiter

If the nodules of a multinodular goiter are not causing symptoms of hyperthyroidism and do not contain cancer, and if the patient has no symptoms, the multinodular goiter is usually left alone.

Doctors used to think that you could shrink a multinodular goiter with thyroid hormone. This has not proven to be the case.

If a patient dislikes the appearance of his or her neck, or if the patient is hyperthyroid, radioactive iodine is used to destroy some of the thyroid tissue (see Chapter 6). This treatment works even for large goiters but sometimes results in hypothyroidism. Also, in the course of destroying thyroid tissue, a lot of thyroid hormone is released into the bloodstream, inducing temporary hyperthyroidism if it isn't present already. Older people, especially, need to receive antithyroid drugs before using radioactive iodine (see Chapter 6).

Some people (less than 10 percent) who are given radioactive iodine to shrink a large multinodular goiter develop Graves' disease, which is discussed in Chapter 6. This complication happens because tissue is released into the blood stream, and the body forms antibodies against it.

Surgery is very rarely done for multinodular goiter unless a cancer is found. Radioactive iodine is able to treat most of these thyroid glands, even the large ones that grow in a downward direction. If surgery is done for a benign multinodular goiter, enough thyroid tissue is left to keep the patient functionally normal. Thyroid hormone pills are not given. Even if they were given, they wouldn't prevent such a gland from growing again.

A patient with a multinodular goiter should return to his or her doctor at least annually to have an examination of the thyroid, or earlier when new growth is seen or pain develops.

Part III
Managing Your Thyroid

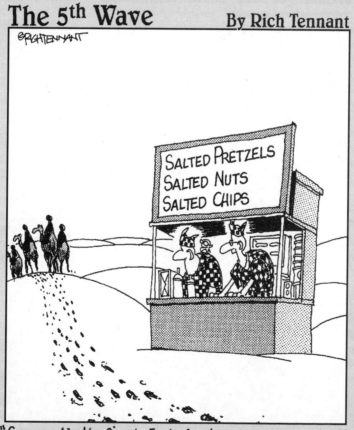

The 5th Wave   By Rich Tennant

©RICHTENNANT

SALTED PRETZELS
SALTED NUTS
SALTED CHIPS

"Go on, that's fine! Just don't come running back yelling 'iodine deficiency'!"

In this part . . .

These chapters clue you into some special situations that can affect your thyroid, particularly infections and medications you take for other conditions. I explain the most prevalent thyroid disorder, iodine deficiency disease. If you must have thyroid surgery, I tell you what to expect and how to prepare. Finally, you discover the genetic link to thyroid diseases and what scientists are doing to try to prevent their transmission from one generation to the next.

Chapter 10

Drugs That Impact Your Thyroid

. . . .

In This Chapter

▶ Realizing the scope of the issue

▶ Knowing the effects of specific drugs

▶ Avoiding drug interactions

▶ Determining whether you are taking one of these drugs

. . . .

*I*t should come as no surprise that a ton of drugs are going to have some effect on your thyroid, because thyroid hormones affect every cell in your body. Drug scientists have not yet reached the stage where they can produce a drug that hits only the target at which they are aiming without banging a few other, unexpected targets along the way. These undesired hits are the *side effects,* and they must be understood so that changes in your thyroid hormone levels or your metabolism that result from using these drugs don't lead to wrong conclusions about the state of your thyroid health.

Certain drugs in our food and in the environment also change thyroid function. These substances, too, need to be understood and perhaps avoided.

Whether you have high blood pressure or a headache or heart failure, at some point you're bound to run into drugs that impact your thyroid function. In this chapter, you meet most of the important drugs that interact with your thyroid in one way or another. If you absorb the information in this chapter, you can probably tell your doctor a thing or two. Try not to embarrass him or her.

Revealing the Drug–Food–Thyroid Connection

Natasha Smart is a 36-year-old woman who is healthy and wants to avoid having any more children. She asks her gynecologist to put her on oral contraceptive tablets. One day, while browsing in a bookstore, she comes upon Dr. Rubin's *tome* (definition: "a scholarly work"), *Thyroid For Dummies.* (She can't miss it; it's featured in the "Must Read" section of the bookstore.) She opens it and reads on the Cheat Sheet at the front of the book that thyroid testing is advised for people over age 35, every 5 years. After buying several copies of the book for herself and her friends, she returns to her gynecologist and asks to be tested.

Her gynecologist, unfortunately, has not read the book and still tests thyroid function with a total thyroxine test (see Chapter 4). The result is high. He tells Natasha that she may have hyperthyroidism. Natasha, proving that her name fits, reads further in the book and finds that the estrogen in oral contraceptive pills raises the amount of thyroid-binding protein in her system. Meanwhile, the *free thyroxine,* the form of the thyroid hormone that can enter cells and, therefore, have an effect, remains normal. She informs her (embarrassed) gynecologist, who does a free T4 test and a TSH (thyroid-stimulating hormone) test, both of which are normal. Nothing further is done.

Leonard Bright is a 72-year-old man who is having trouble with a very irregular heartbeat. His physician places him on a relatively new drug to correct irregular heartbeats called *amiodarone.* About two months later, Leonard's heartbeat has become regular, but he is beginning to feel cold and sleepy. He has gained a few pounds and notices that his skin is dry. His doctor recognizes the symptoms of hypothyroidism (see Chapter 5), sometimes associated with amiodarone. The doctor orders thyroid function tests to confirm the diagnosis and starts Leonard on thyroid hormone. In a month, he has returned to his normal state of health.

Dr. Rubin has followed Kathy Brilliant for many years because of a multinodular goiter. No treatment has been necessary. At the age of 68, she develops a rapid heartbeat and sees a cardiologist. She is placed on amiodarone (the same medication that Mr. Bright takes), and her heart problem resolves. However, after six weeks, she notices that her heart is beating rapidly again. Not only that, she is losing weight and having trouble sleeping. She feels warm all the time although she is well past her menopause.

Kathy returns to the cardiologist, who recognizes that her symptoms are a side effect of amiodarone and sends her back to Dr. Rubin. He tells Kathy that she has hyperthyroidism due to the effect of amiodarone on her multinodular goiter. He suggests that she take pills to control the thyroid and stop taking the amiodarone if the cardiologist can substitute another drug.

Kathy stops the amiodarone and takes pills called *methimazole,* but her condition does not improve. After two months, Dr. Rubin recommends thyroid surgery. When the surgery is done, Kathy improves dramatically. She is now able to take the amiodarone and feels fine.

George Shrub absolutely loves broccoli and consumes prodigious quantities, even at breakfast. He finds that he is often sleepy and cold. He has trouble thinking and making appropriate decisions. He goes to his doctor, who runs blood tests that show a high TSH. The doctor tells George that he is hypothyroid and puts him on thyroid medication.

One night, George and his wife invite Natasha Smart and her husband to dinner. As Natasha watches George consume huge quantities of broccoli, she remarks that she has read in Dr. Rubin's book that broccoli contains a substance that reduces thyroid function. George is very surprised to hear this news, but he sharply reduces his broccoli intake after that night. After talking the situation over with his doctor, he also gradually reduces his thyroid hormone replacement. After he's been off the broccoli for a month, George's thyroid tests are normal.

These cases illustrate the broad spectrum of effects that various drugs and foods can have on thyroid function. Some drugs affect thyroid function tests while the thyroid itself is still normal. Other drugs can create hypothyroidism or hyperthyroidism. As if these effects aren't confusing enough, the same drug given to two different people may cause opposite effects, depending upon their particular clinical situation.

Each year, all the various drug companies get together to produce a huge book called the *Physicians' Desk Reference.* The purpose of this book is to provide, in one convenient place, current information about all the drugs that require prescriptions (a separate book covers nonprescription drugs). Every physician receives a copy of the "PDR" annually. The edition for the year 2000 contains more than 3,500 pages, describing more than 2,000 drugs. It is not an exaggeration to write that most of these drugs affect the thyroid in one way or another. Fortunately, in most cases, the effect is nothing to worry about. But plenty of drugs are a source of concern.

Do I know all the details about how each of these 2,000-plus drugs affects the thyroid? No way, Renee! But I know about the ones that you use most frequently and the ones that have the greatest effect on thyroid function or thyroid function tests. These are the products I discuss in this chapter. I deal with them in terms of how they affect thyroid function.

At the end of the chapter, I group these drugs according to their main clinical purpose so that you can check if you need to be concerned about your blood pressure pill or the pill you take for diabetes or fluid retention. Although I use only the generic (nontrademarked) name in the earlier sections, I give you all the various drug company names at the end of the chapter so you can recognize the particular drug you are taking. For example, *nifedipine* is the generic name for Adalat, Procardia, and Nifedipine Capsules, all the same drug made by different manufacturers. Pretty confusing, huh?

How drugs affect your thyroid hormones

Chapter 3 explains how thyroid hormones are made and released, how they are carried around the body, how they are taken up by cells where they do their work, and how they work within the cells. Drugs can affect thyroid function at any one or more of these levels.

Thyroid hormone is formed when iodine is added to a compound called *thyronine*. When four iodine molecules are attached to this compound, the result is *thyroxine* (T4). When three molecules of iodine are attached, the compound produced is *triiodothyronine* (T3). T3 can also be produced by removing one iodine molecule from thyroxine. Many drugs and food substances block the production of both T4 and T3.

After T3 and T4 are produced, they must travel in the body to get to their site of action. They are carried in the blood stream by thyroid-binding proteins (see Chapter 3). Drugs can affect thyroid function by increasing or decreasing the amount of binding protein in the blood. In this case, thyroid test results can be impacted even while the thyroid function remains normal. This occurs because the *free thyroid hormone* (hormone not bound to protein) is active in the body, not the hormone that is attached to protein.

The free hormone arrives at the cell where it needs to do its work. It must get into the cell by attaching to a substance called a *receptor* on the membrane of the cell. The receptor is another place where certain drugs can prevent thyroid hormone from doing its job. They can block the receptors so that no hormone can enter. The situation may be almost like diabetes, in which plenty of glucose (sugar) is available in the bloodstream for energy, but it can't enter the cell where it does its work.

Once inside the cell, the thyroid hormone attaches to the nucleus, where the genetic material is stored. It then encourages a certain action to take place within that cell. Here, various drugs can block the hormone's attachment to the nucleus or alter it so that it does not produce the desired effect.

Having said this, you should know that new medications come on the market at least hourly. These products get better and better at curing the latest diseases, but their other effects are rarely known from the few thousand people who test them before they come to market. The side effects of many drugs do not become clear until hundreds of thousands of people have taken them. Many if not all of these new drugs affect the thyroid in one way or another. The people who must pay particular attention are those who have some underlying thyroid disease to begin with. For example:

- ✔ If you have had hyperthyroidism (see Chapter 6) and it is under control with antithyroid drugs, a drug containing a lot of iodine will probably cause a recurrence of your disease.

- ✔ If you have had a multinodular goiter (see Chapter 9), iodine will possibly bring on hyperthyroidism.

- ✔ If you are borderline hypothyroid (see Chapter 5), iodine or one of the drugs that block thyroid hormone production will bring on clinical hypothyroidism.

✔ If you have mild subacute thyroiditis (see Chapter 11), some drugs will make it worse to the point that you are symptomatic (that is, you experience symptoms).

Identifying the Effects of Specific Substances

In this section, you encounter particular drugs that affect the thyroid. I group them together according to their potential impact on your thyroid. I don't provide brand names of medications here — only generic names. If you're wondering whether your specific brand of medication is something that may affect your thyroid, check out the listings later in the chapter, where I group these drugs according to their primary purpose.

Initiating or aggravating hypothyroidism

Many drugs have the potential to cause or intensify hypothyroidism. In the following sections, I introduce you to the most commonly prescribed medications that have these potential side effects.

Drugs that compete with iodine

If iodine can't enter the thyroid, thyroid hormone can't be made, and you experience hypothyroidism. Some drugs compete with iodine for entry into the thyroid. Usually the effect is mild, and hypothyroidism doesn't occur. But if your diet is limited in iodine, these drugs can cause low thyroid function. The most important drugs in this category include:

✔ **Lithium,** used for manic-depressive psychosis. In one study, as many as 10 percent of patients given lithium became hypothyroid. This effect is much more common in women than in men and occurs within the first two years of treatment. Most likely, the large population of women with autoimmune thyroid disease (see Chapter 5) is most susceptible to the antithyroid effect of lithium. Not only does lithium block the uptake of iodine, but it also inhibits the production and release of thyroid hormone. Some people being treated with lithium develop a goiter. Curiously (and rarely), lithium can cause hyperthyroidism rather than hypothyroidism.

✔ **Ethionamide,** used in the treatment of tuberculosis. The hypothyroidism that results may or may not be accompanied by goiter.

Minerals such as **fluorine,** which is found in the diet (especially in fluoridated water), have a similar effect on the thyroid. If you consume substantial amounts of fluorine, your thyroid will decrease its production of T4. Your pituitary gland then makes more TSH to stimulate the thyroid, and you could end up with a goiter.

Drugs that prevent the addition of iodine to form thyroid hormones

Another large group of medications blocks the production of thyroid hormones in a slightly different way. They keep iodine from combining with thyronine to form either T4 or T3, the two thyroid hormones. This group of medications includes the following:

- **Aminoglutethimide,** used for the treatment of breast and prostate cancer. As many as one-third of patients treated with this medication develop hypothyroidism.

- **Ketoconazole,** used as an antifungal drug. Hypothyroidism is a rare side effect of this agent.

- **Para-aminosalicylic acid,** used for the long-term treatment of tuberculosis.

- **Sulfonamide drugs,** which eliminate excess water from the body and act as antibiotics. These include **sulfadiazine, sulfasoxazole,** and **acetazoleamide.** If you use these diuretics and antibiotics for prolonged periods of time, they can cause hypothyroidism.

- Certain **sulfonylureas** that are used in the treatment of diabetes, such as **tolbutamide** and **chlorpropamide.** These drugs are rarely used today.

- The **thionamide drugs,** including **propylthiouricil, methimazole,** and **carbimazole.** With the exception of carbimazole, these drugs are discussed extensively in Chapter 6 because they are the primary drugs used to treat hyperthyroidism. Carbimazole is used in the United Kingdom, especially.

Two chemicals found in food have an impact similar to the medications in the preceding list. They are

- **Isoflavins,** found in soybeans. Children fed on large amounts of soy products may develop a goiter.

- **Thiocyanate,** which is contained in many common foods like Brussels sprouts, cauliflower, cabbage, horseradish, kale, kohlrabi, mustard, rutabaga, and turnips. If cattle consume foods like these and you drink milk from those cattle, your thyroid can be affected as well.

Drugs that affect the transport of thyroid hormone

Many drugs affect how thyroid hormones are transported in your bloodstream. Chances are you'll take one of these drugs at some point in your life. If you have normal thyroid function, your thyroid simply makes more or less thyroid hormone to compensate for the effects of these drugs. But if you are hypothyroid and taking a thyroid hormone replacement, your dose may need to be increased or decreased if you have to take one of these drugs.

The following drugs increase thyroid-binding protein, resulting in an increase in total (but not free) thyroxine unless you get your thyroid hormone as a medication:

- ✔ **Estrogens** are the most commonly used drugs in this category. For years, estrogens caused confusion with respect to thyroid function because doctors used to measure how much total thyroxine was in your system, not just how much free thyroxine is there (see Chapter 4). Estrogens are found in birth control pills and hormone replacement therapy. Some animals are fed estrogens to fatten them up, so as you consume those animals, you get estrogen that way as well. The list of medications that contain estrogens is huge.

- ✔ **Clofibrate** is a drug used for lowering blood fats.

- ✔ **Perphenazine** is a treatment for psychotic disorders in the group of drugs called *phenothiazines*. This group includes a number of well-known medications such as **prochlorperazine, trifluoperazine,** and **chlorpromazine.** Perphenazine is the main ingredient in a number of different preparations and is also used for treating nausea and vomiting.

The following drugs decrease thyroid-binding protein resulting in a decrease in total (but not free) thyroxin unless you get your thyroid hormone as a medication:

- ✔ **Anabolic steroids** are used to promote weight gain after extensive surgery or severe illness, as well as in the treatment of anemia. They are rarely used because they frequently cause liver abnormalities.

- ✔ **Androgens** substitute for the male hormone, testosterone, when the patient cannot make his own. They permit muscle growth and normal sexual function.

- ✔ **Glucocorticoids** are used very extensively to treat inflammation and to reduce immunity when the inflammation and autoimmunity are damaging to the body, such as in rheumatoid arthritis and many other illnesses. The list of glucocorticoids is a long one.

- ✔ **Nicotinic acid** is a vitamin used for the treatment of elevated fats in the blood.

If you are hypothyroid and are put on one of these agents for a long time, have your doctor check your thyroid function with a TSH test periodically.

The opiates **heroin** and **methadone** also impact the movement of thyroid hormones in the bloodstream.

Amiodarone

Amiodarone is used for disturbances of the heart rhythm. This drug may cause hypothyroidism in up to 10 percent of the people who take it. The drug is also associated with a number of other side effects, including skin and corneal discoloration and fibrosis of the lungs. It may cause hepatitis and bone marrow suppression. Despite all these negatives, it is very useful in treating heart rhythm disturbances.

Drugs used to treat severe hyperthyroidism

The drugs in this group are very useful when a patient has severe hyperthyroidism and needs to reduce the T3 hormone level as soon as possible. However, these drugs have other primary purposes, and when they are prescribed for those other purposes (to patients who aren't hyperthyroid), they can create hypothyroidism.

- ✔ **Glucocorticoids** are discussed in the previous section.

- ✔ **Iodinated contrast agents** are used for achieving better X-ray studies. Such agents as **ipodate** and **iopanoic acid** have been used in the treatment of hyperthyroidism. A single dose can last for ten days.

- ✔ **Propranolol** is used to slow a rapid heartbeat, but it's also used to treat hyperthyroidism because it controls many of the symptoms, such as palpitations, shakiness, and nervousness.

- ✔ **Propylthiouricil** is one of the standard drugs for the treatment of hyperthyroidism.

Growth hormone

When the body does not make its own growth hormone, an injectable growth hormone restores growth. Growth hormone is administered to children who are not growing properly because they lack this hormone. If someone is borderline hypothyroid, this hormone may push her into hypothyroidism by reducing the T4 hormone to abnormally low levels.

Drugs that remove thyroid hormone from your system

A number of drugs act upon the liver to speed up the metabolism of thyroid hormones into products that are not active. Other drugs pull thyroid hormones out of the body with bowel movements. These drugs are very common.

If you are taking a thyroid replacement hormone and you use one of these drugs, you may develop hypothyroidism. Ask your doctor to check your thyroid hormone levels about a month after you start to take one of these drugs:

- ✔ **Aluminum hydroxide** is used by patients with peptic ulcers to neutralize the acid.

- ✔ **Carbamazepine** and **diphenylhydantoin** are used to treat convulsions.

- ✔ **Cholestyramine** and **colestipol** are used to reduce fats.

- ✔ **Ferrous sulfate** is given to people who are deficient in iron and have anemia. At some point, the ferrous sulfate treatment is stopped when the patient's iron reserves are full. The patient may actually become hyperthyroid at that point, if her thyroid hormone dose was increased due to the initial effects of the drug.

- ✔ **Phenobarbital** is used for the treatment of convulsions as well as for mild anxiety.

- ✔ **Rifampin** is one of the treatments for tuberculosis. This drug very rarely causes hypothyroidism in a person who takes thyroid hormone.

- ✔ **Sucralfate** is used for peptic ulcer disease. It may result in hypothyroidism if it's taken chronically.

It is important to monitor your thyroid function both during and after use of a short-term medication that lowers the levels of thyroid hormone in your blood, especially if you are taking oral thyroid medication.

Drugs that decrease your TSH

The following drugs can lower the level of thyroid-stimulating hormone in your system, potentially leading to lower thyroid function:

- ✔ **Acetylsalicylic acid** is commonly known as aspirin. People taking more than 8 or 10 aspirin daily might suffer this effect on TSH.

- ✔ **Bromergocryptine** is given to prevent lactation (milk production) and to shrink prolactin-secreting pituitary tumors.

- ✔ **Clofibrate** is given to lower the fat particles that contain triglycerides. It also lowers the TSH but doesn't seem to cause clinical problems.

- ✔ **Dopamine** is used to lower blood pressure, especially in an emergency setting. It lowers TSH but is not usually used long enough to cause problems with hypothyroidism.

- ✔ **Glucocorticoids** are used to treat inflammation and reduce immunity.

- ✔ **Octreotide** is a drug that treats certain tumors that produce hormones, especially *acromegaly,* which produces excessive growth hormone, and *carcinoid tumors,* which produce a chemical that causes severe diarrhea and flushing.

- ✔ **Opiates,** including morphine and heroin, are used legally for pain control and illegally for a chemical high.

- ✔ **Phentolamine** is given to control blood pressure in a patient who has a tumor of the adrenal gland called a *pheochromocytoma*. It reduces TSH but is not generally given long enough to make a difference in thyroid function.

- **Pyridoxine** is vitamin B6. It is given during pregnancy and when there is evidence that someone has this vitamin deficiency.

- **Thyroid hormones** are given to replace a deficiency or to suppress thyroid cancer or a goiter. They suppress the production of TSH.

Creating false test results

Certain drugs can alter the thyroid hormone (T3 and T4) tests that measure total thyroid hormones (but not free thyroid hormones, which remain normal). If you're taking one of the drugs listed here, you and your doctor should keep that fact in mind if your total T4 test shows hypothyroidism but you aren't experiencing any symptoms of the condition.

- **Salicylates** such as aspirin are the most commonly used drugs in this group.

- **Diphenylhydantoin** and **carbamazepine** are used as treatment for convulsions.

- **Furosemide** causes the loss of excess water through the kidneys.

- **Heparin** is used to prevent blood clots. It doesn't change your thyroid function, but if you are given an injection of *low molecular weight heparin,* a measurement of free T4 taken within 10 hours of the injection will be falsely elevated.

- **Orphenadrine** is used in a number of drug preparations for the relief of muscle spasms. It is not a muscle relaxant but may reduce pain.

Causing an increase in thyroid activity

The following drugs increase the production of TSH, which can result in hyperthyroidism:

- **Amphetamine** is used to reduce congestion and is also used (inappropriately) as a weight loss agent.

- **Cimetidine** and **ranitidine** are used to reduce acid secretion to treat peptic ulcers. Both can raise the TSH, but studies don't show a change in thyroid function with these drugs.

- **Clomiphene** brings on ovulation to promote pregnancy. It has effects on several of the hormones in the pituitary gland, including TSH.

- **L-dopa inhibitors** such as **chlorpromazine** and **haloperidol** are used in the management of psychotic disorders. They have been shown to raise TSH, although the patients do not generally become hyperthyroid.

✔ **Metoclopramide** and **domperidone** are used to control nausea and vomiting, especially after surgery. Metoclopramide is also used for gastrointestinal disorders in diabetes mellitus.

✔ **Iodine** can raise TSH levels as it blocks the release of thyroid hormones.

✔ **Lithium** raises TSH, in addition to all its other effects on thyroid function. In very rare cases, it can cause hyperthyroidism. (It causes hypothyroidism much more frequently.)

Preventing Harmful Drug Interactions

With so many drugs having an effect on thyroid function in one way or another, it becomes very difficult to avoid drug interactions, particularly if one of the drugs you're taking is thyroid hormone. If you're taking thyroid hormone, it means that your body isn't able to make the subtle changes in thyroid function necessary to compensate for the other drug you're taking, which is most likely reducing the thyroid hormone available to your systems.

The best solution is to ask your doctor either to run a program on his computer that looks at multiple drugs and determines interactions or to have your druggist do the same thing. If the doctor doesn't have the capability to do this check, he can ask his hospital pharmacy to do it.

Discovering Whether You Are at Risk

You may not recognize many of the drugs named in the previous sections, because I've used their generic names. The generic name is the official name of the drug regardless of the name the manufacturer gives it.

In this section, I list brand names of these drugs, and I group them according to their usage. If you have a specific medical problem — for example, high blood pressure — go to that section, look at the drugs listed there, and see whether the brand name is the same as the one you're using.

If one of the drugs listed here is something you take, it may be a good idea to ask your doctor to run thyroid function tests.

Anemia drugs

Ferrous sulfate: Feosol Elixer and Tablets, Fero-Folic 500 Filmtab Tablets, Fero-Grad 500 Filmtab Tablets, Iberet-500 Liquid and Tablets, Irospan Capsules and Tablets, Slow Fe Tablets, Fe-50 Caplets, Vi-Daylin/F Multivitamin and Iron Drops With Floride

Antiaddiction agents

Methadone: Dolophine Hydrochloride Tablets, Methadone HCl Powder, Methadose Dispersible Tablets, Methadose Oral Tablets

Antibiotics

Ethionamide: Trecator-SC Tablets

Ketoconazole: Nizoral Tablets, Ketoconazole Tablets

Para-aminosalicylic acid: Paser Granules

Sulfonamide drugs: Bactrim Tablets, Septra Tablets

Rifampin: Rifadin Capsules, Rifater

Anti-inflammatory drugs

Glucocorticoids: Celestone, Decadron, Depo-Medrol, Hydrocortone Tablets, Solu-medrol Sterile Powder

Aspirin: Darvon Compound, Ecotrin Enteric Coated Aspirin, Excedrin, Fiorinal Halprin Tablets, Norgesic Tablets, Percodan Tablets, Robaxisal Tablets, Soma Compound, Fiortal Capsules, Gelpirin Tablets, Propoxyphene Compound, Roxiprin Tablets

Antithyroid drugs

Propylthiouricil: Propylthiouricil Tablets

Methimazole: Tapazol Tablets, Methimazole Tablets

Control growth hormone

Octreotide: Sandostatin

Control nausea

Metoclopramide: Reglan, Metoclopramide Tablets

Control prolactin

Bromergocryptine: Parlodel Capsules, Bromocryptine Mesylate Tablets

Diabetes drugs

Tolbutamide: Orinase

Chlorpropamide: Diabinase

Diuretics (reduce body water)

Furosemide: Lasix, Furosemide Tablets

Drugs to improve alertness

Amphetamine: Adderall Tablets

Fat-lowering drugs

Clofibrate: Atromid-S Capsules

Cholestyramine: LoCholest Powder, Questran Light for Oral Suspension, Prevalite for Oral Suspension

Colestipol: Colestid Tablets

Heart rhythm drugs

Amiodarone: Cardarone Tablets, Pacerone Tablets

Propranolol: Inderal Tablets, Propranolol HCl Tablets

Phentolamine: Regitine Vials

Hormone replacement

Estrogens (female hormones): Estinyl Tablets, Estrace Vaginal Cream, Estratab Tablets, Menest Tablets, Ogen Tablets, Premarin Tablets, Vagifem Tablets

Estrogen and Progestin Combinations: Activella Tablets, Brevicon 28-Day Tablets, Demulen (many strengths), Desogen Tablets, Estrostep 21 Tablets, Levora Tablets, Lo/Ovral Tablets, Mircette Tablets, Modicon Tablets, Necon Tablets (many strengths), Norinyl Tablets (many strengths), Ortho Tri-Cyclen Tablets (many strengths), Ortho-Cyclen Tablets (many strengths), Ortho-Novum Tablets (many strengths), Ovcon Tablets, Premphase Tablets, Prempro Tablets, Trinorinyl-28 Tablets, Triphasil Tablets, Trivora Tablets, Zovia Tablets

Anabolic steroids: Anandrol-50 Tablets, Oxandrin Tablets, Winstrol Tablets

Androgens (male hormones): Androderm Transdermal System, AndroGel, Android Capsules, Delatestryl Injection, Testoderm Transdermal Systems, Testred Capsules

Growth Hormone: Geref for Injection, Humatrope, Nutropin, Protropin, Saizen for Injection

Clomiphene: Clomid Tablets, Serophene Tablets, Clomiphene Citrate Tablets

Thyroid hormones: Synthroid, Levothroid, Levoxyl Tablets

Pain medication

Morphine: Astramorph/PF Injection, Duramorpf Injection, Kadian Capsules, MS Contin Tablets, MSIR Oral Capsules, Oramorph SR Tablets, Roxanol 100 Concentrated Oral Solution, Morphine Sulfate, OMS Concentrate CII, RMS Suppositories CII

Peptic ulcer drugs

Aluminum hydroxide: Amphogel, Maalox, Mylanta, Alu-Cap Capsules, Alumina and Magnesia Oral Suspension

Sucralfate: Carafate Suspension and Tablets, Sucralfate Tablets

Cimetidine: Tagamet, Cimetidine Tablets

Ranitidine: Zantac, Ranitidine HCl

Psychoactive drugs

Lithium: Eskalith Capsules, Eskalith CR Controlled Release Tablets, Lithium Carbonate Capsules, Lithobid Slow-Release Tablets

Perphenazine: Estrafon 2-10 Tablets, Estrafon Tablets, Estrafon-Forte Tablets, Trilafon Tablets, Perphenazine Tablets

Chlorpromazine: Thorazine, Chlorpromazine HCl

Haloperidol: Haldol

Chapter 11

Thyroid Infections and Inflammation

In This Chapter

▶ Encountering subacute thyroiditis

▶ Dealing with postpartum and silent thyroiditis

▶ Suffering from acute thyroiditis

▶ Finding out about more rare forms of thyroiditis

The term *thyroiditis* is used in this book (see Chapter 5) to denote the most common form of apparent inflammation of the thyroid, autoimmune thyroiditis, also known as Hashimoto's thyroiditis and chronic thyroiditis. In this chapter, I introduce you to causes of thyroiditis that are less common than autoimmune disorders but just as important to know about. Usually, but not always, thyroiditis is associated with infection.

Fortunately, infection of the thyroid is rare, perhaps because of all the iodine and hydrogen peroxide in the thyroid gland. If you ever had a boo-boo when you were young, your mother probably covered it with a solution containing iodine or hydrogen peroxide, both of which kill bugs.

Despite all this natural protection, every so often people develop an infected thyroid. In this chapter, you discover how doctors tell one form of infection from another, as well as the method of treatment and the prognosis for each illness.

Putting a Face on Subacute Thyroiditis

Joan Sharp is a 40-year-old woman who has been suffering from a cold and a cough with a low-grade fever for about a week. One morning, she awakens and notices that her neck hurts. She can tell that the pain is located in the center of her neck beneath her Adam's apple. She goes to her doctor, who notes that her thyroid is enlarged and tender. The doctor also finds that Joan is nervous, and her fingers are shaking slightly.

Dr. Hammerbe sends Joan to the lab for some tests. The lab results show that her free T4 is elevated while her TSH is depressed (see Chapter 4), suggesting hyperthyroidism. The doctor does a test for inflammation called an *erythrocyte sedimentation rate,* and the result is elevated. Knowing that neck pain is unusual in hyperthyroidism due to Grave's disease (see Chapter 6), Dr. Hammerbe calls Dr. Rubin about what to do next.

Dr. Rubin suggests that she do a blood test for *serum thyroglobulin,* which comes back high, and a thyroid uptake (see Chapter 4), which comes back low. Joan finds out that she has subacute thyroiditis. She is started on aspirin and rapidly improves. The swelling of her neck declines, and the tenderness rapidly decreases.

Causes and effects

Subacute thyroiditis has gone by many names in the past, including *De Quervain's thyroiditis, giant cell thyroiditis,* and *subacute painful thyroiditis.* It is called *subacute* to differentiate it from the condition I discuss later in the chapter, *acute* thyroiditis, which is usually much more painful and associated with more symptoms that make the patient sick.

Subacute thyroiditis is not very common. In my practice, which is about 60 percent diabetes mellitus and 40 percent thyroid disease, I see perhaps two cases per year.

As you can tell from the case of Joan Sharp, this condition often begins with an infection that suggests a virus. The person may have muscle aches and fever, and then begins to feel neck pain in the area of the thyroid. This pain may be severe. The neck pain usually brings the patient to the doctor. When the doctor examines the patient, the thyroid is not only painful but enlarged as well.

Evidence exists that subacute thyroiditis may be caused by a virus: Cases of this condition tend to be seasonal, and they sometimes occur in outbreaks like any infectious disease. Over the years, doctors have looked for a particular virus that might be the cause of all cases of subacute thyroiditis, but no one virus has ever been isolated in all cases. The only virus that has been found with some frequency is the mumps virus.

Subacute thyroiditis seems to occur more often in people who have decreased immunity from infection, such as AIDS patients or people who are getting bone marrow transplants for leukemia.

As a result of the inflammation, the thyroid releases much of its stored hormone along with the stored thyroglobulin (see Chapter 4). The virus seems to temporarily damage thyroid cells at this point. The large quantity of released thyroid hormone produces hyperthyroidism. Because the thyroid cells are damaged and the production of thyroid hormone isn't ongoing, the hyperthyroidism lasts only a brief time, sometimes a few days, until the thyroid gland is depleted of hormone. The patient goes through a brief period of normal thyroid function as hormone levels fall, and then swings into the opposite condition, hypothyroidism. Finally, because a viral illness usually doesn't last, the thyroid gland returns to normal, the pain goes away, and the thyroid function returns to normal.

Like most thyroid conditions, subacute thyroiditis is more common in women than men; the ratio of cases is 3 to 1. This condition appears to have some genetic basis because the same genetic marker — an antigen on human white blood cells — is found in about 75 percent of cases, suggesting that these patients are more susceptible to the disease because of their genetic makeup. In fact, two different genetic markers have been described. Each one seems to be associated with the disease occurring at a different time of the year, although in either case it generally occurs in the fourth or fifth decade of life.

There's a small (about two percent) but definite possibility of a recurrence some years later. This will generally be milder than the original attack. Occasionally, a patient may experience repeated attacks of pain. Thyroid hormone will help to prevent such recurrences, but if recurrences aren't prevented, it's necessary to remove the thyroid with surgery or radioactive iodine.

Laboratory findings

Lab tests are very helpful in pinning down a diagnosis of subacute thyroiditis. Some of the findings are as follows:

- The *erythrocyte sedimentation rate,* a general blood test for inflammation, is often unusually high considering the relative mildness of the symptoms, sometimes reaching a value of over 100, when the normal is about 20.

- Shortly after the thyroid becomes infected, up to 50 percent of patients experience hyperthyroidism, so TSH level are low while FT4 levels are elevated.

- The inflammation causes the release of a large quantity of both T4 and T3. Because the thyroid contains so much more T4 relative to T3, compared to the blood, there's a drop in the ratio of T4 to T3 as they escape into the blood stream.

- If liver tests are done, the level of *alkaline phosphatase* is often elevated. It appears that the infection affects the liver in addition to the thyroid, though the impact on the liver is mild.

✔ Blood tests show that a lot of thyroglobulin is present in the blood.

✔ The test for thyroid autoantibodies (see Chapter 4) is negative.

✔ Some specialists suggest that a thyroid ultrasound study (see Chapter 4) is distinctive in subacute thyroiditis, but this test is not usually done.

✔ The key test, the thyroid uptake of radioactive iodine, is very low, which differentiates this condition from other causes of hyperthyroidism.

When the results of all these tests and the clinical picture are put together, the diagnosis is fairly certain, although no one test proves that subacute thyroiditis is present. To prove the diagnosis, a biopsy of the gland is necessary, but the mildness of the disease means that a biopsy rarely needs to be done.

Subacute thyroiditis is differentiated from other forms of thyroiditis by the presence of generalized thyroid pain, though sometimes the pain may occur on one side of the thyroid only. Another cause of a painful thyroid is bleeding, producing a hemorrhagic thyroid cyst. This pain usually occurs on one side of the thyroid and is not preceded by a viral illness. Lab tests help to secure a diagnosis, particularly a radioactive uptake, which is normal for the cystic thyroid but low for subacute thyroiditis. In rare cases, chronic thyroiditis is painful (see Chapter 5). With chronic thyroiditis, levels of thyroid autoantibodies are high.

Treatment options

At the beginning of subacute thyroiditis, when the patient is hyperthyroid, a drug such as propranolol can be used to reverse the symptoms of excessive thyroid hormone. (Propranolol is a beta blocker that slows the heart, decreases anxiety, and reduces tremor.) Antithyroid drugs like propylthiouricil and methimazole have no place in this treatment, because the thyroid is not chronically making excessive hormones.

The thyroid pain can be managed with aspirin or a nonsteroidal anti-inflammatory agent. Once in a while it's necessary to use a steroid like prednisone for a week or two. When the uptake of radioactive iodine returns to normal, the inflammation is finished, and steroids can be stopped.

With the end of symptoms, the patient is back to normal permanently in almost every case. Like so much in medicine, there are rare exceptions where the disease goes away and then returns or the pain is persistent. These patients may need to have their thyroids removed to finally control the disease.

Coping with Postpartum and Silent Thyroiditis

Michelle Clever is a 29-year-old woman who gave birth to a healthy boy about five months ago. Recently she has noticed that her neck is larger than before, but it's not painful. She is feeling nervous, and her hands shake. She has trouble going to sleep, which makes her situation tough because the baby wakes her up at night. She can feel her heart beating rapidly at times.

Michelle goes to her obstetrician, who examines her and tells her that she is probably hyperthyroid. She is sent to see Dr. Rubin, who notes that she was pregnant recently. He obtains thyroid function tests, which are elevated. Dr. Rubin tells Michelle that he believes she probably has postpartum thyroiditis. He places her on the beta blocker propranolol, which controls her symptoms well. He also explains that she will probably go through a phase of low thyroid function before she returns to normal. A few weeks later she appears to be better.

Several weeks after that, Michelle notices that she is feeling cold and having trouble keeping awake. Dr. Rubin reassures her that this is the hypothyroid phase of postpartum thyroiditis. Within a few weeks, she feels normal. Two years later, after a second pregnancy, the problem recurs.

Understanding the disease

Postpartum and silent thyroiditis are considered to be variations of the same disease. Postpartum thyroiditis occurs usually three to six months after a pregnancy, while silent thyroiditis can happen to anyone at any time.

This disease is considered to be an autoimmune disorder because high levels of peroxidase autoantibodies can be found in the blood (see Chapter 4). In this condition, the antibodies seem to damage thyroid cells, causing a release of thyroid hormone that leads to temporary hyperthyroidism. So far, no single gene has been found to be associated with this form of thyroiditis.

Postpartum thyroiditis is very common; it occurs after 5 to 10 percent of all pregnancies. With this condition, unlike subacute thyroiditis, a patient has no symptoms of fever or weakness, although she may complain of feeling warm. A rapid heartbeat and palpitations are part of the condition. The thyroid itself is not painful, although it's often abnormally large. The changes that occur in thyroid function are similar to those that occur with subacute thyroiditis, however. First there's hyperthyroidism, followed by normal function, followed by hypothyroidism. The hypothyroidism may resolve, but the patient is at high risk for permanent hypothyroidism.

Women who develop postpartum thyroiditis show a high rate of recurrence in later pregnancies, and 25 percent of them are permanently hypothyroid after three to five years. As many as 50 percent are hypothyroid after seven to nine years. The recurrence rate of silent thyroiditis is also very high.

Ten percent of women with postpartum thyroiditis experience depression. Any woman complaining of postpartum depression should be tested for low thyroid function.

Interpreting lab results

The lab test that best distinguishes a patient with subacute thyroiditis from a patient with postpartum or silent thyroiditis is the test of *erythrocyte sedimentation rate*. With subacute thyroiditis, that rate is high, but with postpartum or silent thyroiditis, the rate is normal.

Thyroid function tests from patients with postpartum or silent thyroiditis are initially high, then normal, then low. As in subacute thyroiditis, the hyperthyroid phase of the disease is due to leakage from the thyroid. Because the ratio of T4 to T3 is much higher in the thyroid than it is in the blood, the ratio of T4 to T3 temporarily becomes high in the blood as well. The TSH and the radioactive uptake of iodine are also on the low side during the hyperthyroid phase.

Getting treatment

Treatment for postpartum and silent thyroiditis depends upon the stage at which the disease is diagnosed. If the patient is diagnosed during the hyperthyroid phase, she is given the beta blocker propranolol, which helps to control the symptoms of hyperthyroidism. Antithyroid drugs aren't useful in this case because they won't prevent hyperthyroidism caused by a leakage of thyroid hormone. When the hypothyroidism phase occurs, thyroid hormone replacement is given with the understanding that it may not be needed on a permanent basis.

Identifying Acute Thyroiditis

Patrick Clever is a 45-year-old man who has suddenly developed severe pain in his neck, fever, and chills. The pain is so severe that he has to bend his neck forward to cope with it. He can't swallow without pain. He also feels weak.

Patrick goes off to see his doctor, who notes that he is very sick. His thyroid gland is exquisitely tender, and he has a fever. The doctor sends him to his thyroid specialist friend, Dr. Rubin, who notes that the tender area is somewhat soft. He puts a fine needle into it and removes a quantity of pus. The pus is sent for culture and for staining to determine the bug causing the infection, and Patrick is placed on an antibiotic, along with aspirin.

In a few days, Patrick is feeling much better. The pus grows out a bug that is sensitive to the antibiotic, which is continued for 10 days. Patrick recovers fully.

Acute thyroiditis is much more rare than subacute thyroiditis but can be confused with it, depending upon the way the disease appears in the patient. In my 27 years in practice, I have seen only four cases. However, because many more people have lost their immunity to infection as a result of the AIDS epidemic, doctors will probably see more cases in the near future.

Describing the disease

Many different organisms have been found in the thyroid glands of patients with acute thyroiditis. Bacteria are present about 70 percent of the time. The type of bacteria varies from *pneumococcus* (which often causes pneumonia) to *streptococcus* (associated with strep throat) to *staphylococcus* (which causes skin infections). About 15 percent of the time, a fungus is the infecting organism; tuberculosis is the cause 10 percent of the time, and various other bugs are the culprits much less frequently.

Besides the tender thyroid, nearby structures such as the trachea (voice box) and esophagus (swallowing tube) are inflamed, and local lymph glands in the neck are tender. In many patients, a connection from the outside (such as the throat) to the thyroid tissue is found, through which the infection invades. This connection is called a *fistula* and is a result of abnormal development from birth. It acts as an open pipe to the thyroid for the passage of the infection. If a fistula is found in association with acute thyroiditis, it must be removed or infection will recur. Infection of the thyroid is so rare that a fistula should be looked for in every case.

A patient with acute thyroiditis looks obviously sick. He (or she) complains of the pain in his neck and may have to bend his neck forward to decrease it. He has a fever and chills. The thyroid is enlarged (usually on one side), hot, and tender. Depending on how large the thyroid gets, the patient may have trouble swallowing or even breathing. Lymph nodes are often enlarged, swollen, and tender as well.

Confirming the diagnosis with lab tests

In a patient with acute thyroiditis, general blood tests for infection, such as the white blood count and the erythrocyte sedimentation rate, are abnormally high. These results confirm that an infection or inflammation is present.

When thyroid tests such as the free T4 and the TSH are done, the results are generally normal, although once in a while the destruction of the thyroid is so great that enough hormone leaks to cause hyperthyroidism. Thyroid uptake of radioactive iodine is normal. Thyroid autoantibodies are negative.

The best test for acute thyroiditis is a needle biopsy. Usually the biopsy shows inflammation and the infecting organism, but occasionally, no inflammation is seen. Then the diagnosis is much more difficult. Sometimes the thyroid has an abscess, which is drained by the needle.

Treating acute thyroiditis

The treatment for this condition is to give the appropriate antibiotic based upon the suspected organism. The biopsy can provide a good idea of what type of organism is causing the infection, which can be confirmed by a culture of the biopsy tissue. The right antibiotic generally cures the infection and restores normal thyroid function. Sometimes the infection does not respond, and surgery to remove the infected part of the thyroid or the whole thyroid is necessary.

When acute thyroiditis recurs, a doctor should suspect that a fistula is allowing bugs to get into the thyroid from the outside. In that situation, the patient does a barium swallow, which shows a trail of barium going from the throat into the thyroid gland. Surgery is required to eliminate a fistula.

Occasionally, acute thyroiditis causes such damage to the thyroid tissue that the patient needs to take replacement thyroid hormone.

A Most Rare Form of Thyroiditis

ANECDOTE

Christopher Dull is a 42-year-old man who comes to his doctor complaining of gaining weight and feeling tired, weak, cold, and sleepy. He also says that his neck feels very tight. He has trouble swallowing and breathing.

His doctor examines him and notes that his neck feels very dense. His thyroid barely moves when he swallows. The doctor does not feel swelling in the lymph nodes in his neck.

The doctor runs thyroid function tests, which show a low free T4 and a high TSH. At the same time, he obtains a calcium level, and this test result is low as well. A test of the hormone made by the parathyroid glands called *parathyroid hormone* is run, and the result of that test is low. The doctor sends Chris for a barium swallow, which shows compression on the esophagus. He refers Chris to Dr. Rubin.

Dr. Rubin attempts to do a fine needle biopsy of Chris's thyroid but is unable to get tissue. Dr. Rubin makes a presumptive diagnosis of *Riedel's thyroiditis.* He starts Chris on steroids, thyroid hormone, and calcium. Chris's symptoms gradually decrease, but the hypothyroidism and the *hypoparathyroidism* (low parathyroid function resulting in low calcium) remain. Chris continues to take thyroid hormone replacement and vitamin D for the rest of his life.

To be thorough, I feel that I need to discuss this final form of thyroiditis even though I have seen only one case in my career. The disease is called *Riedel's thyroiditis.* The cause is not known. It is associated with elevated levels of antithyroid autoantibodies so autoimmunity is probably playing some role, especially in view of the good response to steroids. Some specialists believe that Riedel's thyroiditis is a variant of chronic autoimmune thyroiditis (see Chapter 5). Both conditions are associated with autoantibodies and both have been found to have other autoimmune diseases coexisting in the same patient.

Riedel's thyroiditis is said to be twice as frequent in men as in women, but there are so few recorded cases that it's hard to tell. It tends to occur between ages 30 and 60.

What happens to the thyroid is that there is a *fibrosis* — the replacement of thyroid tissue by hard fibers that can be so dense that thyroid function is lost and the patient becomes hypothyroid. The fibrous tissue firmly attaches the thyroid to the trachea and the nearby muscles so that it doesn't move in the neck. A small needle can't penetrate the fibrous thyroid.

If the fibrosis continues, it involves the parathyroid glands, which sit behind the thyroid. They can be destroyed, and the patient develops hypoparathyroidism. Because the parathyroid glands are important for maintaining calcium levels, the result of this disease is a fall in calcium. Symptoms of tingling and numbness in the hands and feet and tingling around the mouth begin to occur. As the calcium falls, it can result in severe muscle spasms.

Sometimes the fibrosis stops and the patient remains stable. Other times it continues, and the patient has trouble breathing, swallowing, and even talking.

When the doctor does thyroid function tests early in the disease, they may be normal. Later the patient becomes hypothyroid. The erythrocyte sedimentation rate is normal as well.

Because the fibrosis can be so invasive, Reidel's thyroiditis is sometimes confused with anaplastic carcinoma, an extremely rapid-growing, invasive form of thyroid cancer that is usually fatal (see Chapter 8). A biopsy generally shows the difference. Sometimes the condition is not recognized until the patient is in the operating room about to have surgery for what is thought to be cancer.

If severe neck symptoms occur, surgery may be necessary to free up the tissues. Sometimes so much fibrosis is present that surgery isn't successful in removing the tissue. A trial of steroids often slows or stops progression of the disease. The other agent that has shown some success is the drug tamoxifen.

Chapter 12

Iodine Deficiency Disease

*I*n the movie *Love and Death,* Woody Allen describes a convention of village idiots in Russia. If such a convention actually occurred, sadly, most of the people in attendance would probably be suffering from iodine deficiency disease.

As you discover in this chapter, iodine deficiency disease is the world's most common and preventable cause of mental retardation. What stops it from being eliminated is more often politics than medicine. The situation is very similar to the problem of infectious diseases that can be prevented with immunization. The science of the condition is clearly understood, including the treatment. What's missing is the means to transfer that knowledge into action.

A case in point is the story of the former East Germany. Prior to 1980, 50 percent of East German adolescents developed goiters. In 1980, the country began a program of adding minute amounts of iodine to common table salt, and the percentage of adolescents with goiter dropped to less than 1 percent. With the reunification of Germany, iodization became voluntary, and the goiter rate began to rise again.

This chapter gives you a greater appreciation of the major role of thyroid hormone in the growth and development of the human body, particularly mental development. When you finish this chapter, you won't have any chance of getting invited to that convention in Russia.

Realizing the Vastness of the Problem

More than one-quarter of the world's population suffers from some level of iodine deficiency disease. That works out to 1.6 billion people. Of these, 655 million have a *goiter,* an enlargement of the thyroid that can sometimes be debilitating. Twenty-six million of them have brain damage, and 6 million of those 26 million are *cretins,* individuals so handicapped by their thyroid conditions that they are completely dependent upon those around them to live. Some researchers believe that for each day we delay treating this vast problem, 50,000 infants are born with decreased mental capacity caused by an iodine deficiency.

The reason so many people suffer is that the food they eat or the ground from which that food comes contains little or no iodine. Chapter 3 explains that iodine is required to form *thyroxine* (T4) and *triiodothyronine* (T3), the two major thyroid hormones.

All soil on earth used to contain iodine. However, over hundreds of thousands of years, the iodine has been leached out of the soil in two major areas of the earth: the high mountains and the plains, far from oceans, that were covered by water in the past. The high mountains were once covered with glaciers. As the glaciers melted, they carried iodine out of the soil, back to the ocean. In the same way, the flooded plains leached iodine from the soil and carried it back to the ocean as the water flowed away. As a result, high mountains and plains far from oceans are the areas where iodine deficiency disease is most often found.

Crops that grow in such soil are iodine deficient. Animals that feed on these crops become iodine deficient. If the animal happens to be a cow that provides milk, children who drink that milk may be iodine deficient. The meat from that cow is also iodine deficient. The result is a huge public health problem. Even pets such as dogs become iodine deficient.

If you looked at a map of the world that shows the areas where iodine deficiency disease is most prevalent, you'd see that vast areas of China, Russia, Mexico, South America, and Africa are rife with the disease. Surprisingly, the United States is not spared. At one time, the iodization of salt and the addition of iodine to bread seemed to solve the problem in the U.S. More recently, as shown in a study in the *Journal of Clinical Endocrinology and Metabolism* in October 1998, Americans have decreased their iodine intake. Nearly 12 percent of those studied had insufficient iodine in their urine. (The urine test is a reliable measurement of daily iodine intake.) This number compares with only 3 percent with insufficient iodine intake 20 years earlier.

Western Europe, also, used to be virtually free from iodine deficiency, but recent studies among Europeans have shown decreases in iodine intake as well.

How iodine deficiency is measured

In order to determine whether iodine deficiency is present in large populations, it was necessary to develop simple tools to measure a lack of iodine. One simple technique is a measurement of iodine in the urine. In areas where iodine is not deficient, the iodine in the urine is 100 micrograms per day or more.

If a country or population undertakes an iodization program, this urine test is taken before the population receives iodine and at intervals afterward to see whether the program is working. (If it is, a much higher level of iodine appears in the urine after iodization begins.)

The second important measure of iodine deficiency is the frequency of goiters. A goiter is said to be present if the lobes of the thyroid are larger than the end parts of the thumbs of the person being examined. (These parts are called the *terminal phalanges* of the thumbs.) Unfortunately, such a measurement of the thyroid is very hard to make in practice, especially in small children where it is most important. To overcome this difficulty, doctors use a portable ultrasound device (see Chapter 4), which produces a measurement that is highly accurate and reproducible.

Finally, measurement of thyroid hormones and TSH in the blood can be performed to evaluate the production of thyroid hormones.

Facing the Consequences of Iodine Lack

If your body lacks iodine, it can't produce sufficient thyroid hormone. This deficiency has severe consequences at every stage of life. This section discusses the price paid in bad health and abnormal function at every stage of life, beginning with the pregnant woman and her fetus.

Pregnancy

Even before pregnancy, a lack of T4 hormone has a harmful effect. Women who are hypothyroid have greater difficulties becoming pregnant, and they have more miscarriages and stillbirths than women with normal thyroid function.

A fetus doesn't begin to make thyroid hormone until the 24th week of pregnancy. Until then, it's dependent upon the mother's T4. During this time, the fetal brain is developing, and the entire chain of events that produces a normal brain requires T4 at every stage. If this hormone is lacking, the consequences are severe.

If a fetus is deficient in T4, its brain triggers an increase in the amount of the enzyme that converts T4 to T3 within the brain. This form of the enzyme is not found in other tissues, so the brain may be protected from hypothyroidism while the rest of the body is not.

The entire body's formation is dependent upon adequate T4. If sufficient hormone is not available, congenital anomalies may occur. The infant may not survive much past birth. If it does, it may not live more than a few years. In this nuclear age, it's important to realize that a thyroid gland that is not making enough thyroid hormone will take up large amounts of iodine from whatever source it can. In the case of a nuclear accident where radioactive iodine is released, a hypothyroid mother will concentrate the iodine and pass it on to her growing fetus. If radioactive iodine does not completely destroy the fetal thyroid, that thyroid will at least be very prone to develop thyroid cancer.

Infancy

A new baby deprived of iodine will have a goiter and show signs of hypothyroidism. Depending upon the severity of the lack, the baby may be a cretin, which I explain later in this chapter. The brain of a newborn continues to develop up to age 2, so providing iodine starting immediately after birth may prevent retardation. A baby lacking in iodine also shows increased susceptibility to radioactive iodine (or any iodine).

Childhood

Iodine-deficient children often have goiters. They show reduced intelligence and poor motor function, and they may be deaf. Like infants, these children have a tendency to accumulate iodine from any source and are at greater risk in the case of a nuclear accident.

Adulthood

After the iodine-deficient child has grown up, a goiter is often present in an iodine-deficient adult, though not always. He or she is intellectually retarded and may have movement difficulties. This person's thyroid gland is highly susceptible to radioactivity.

As you can see, the costs of iodine deficiency disorder are enormous both for the individual and for society. A village filled with people like those described here would not be able to govern itself or provide an economic base to help better the condition of the people, or to take the steps necessary to overcome the problem, including using iodine.

Endemic Cretinism

Shabmir is a 46-year-old woman living in Pakistan. Since she can remember, she has had a huge growth on the front of her neck that the doctors tell her is a goiter. She is not alone, because more than 70 percent of the villagers around her suffer from the same condition.

Shabmir attended the local school but seems to have no aptitude for learning. Because of the unsightly growth on her neck, she has been discriminated against by those who do not have the same problem (perhaps because they come from an area with sufficient iodine in the food). Not only that, but the goiter is so large that she has difficulty moving her head and neck, which makes it hard for her to earn a living. She did not marry until she found another person who had a severe goiter.

For years, Shabmir was unable to become pregnant. When she did, the baby was stillborn. She has not been pregnant again.

She appears swollen and lethargic. She has very little interest in her neighbors or her surroundings, and she tends to sleep a lot.

Shabmir's story is typical of the way that iodine deficiency disease affects the lives of millions of people. It's a worldwide plague that can render whole populations unable to function. The shame is that this condition is completely preventable!

In this section, I show you the different ways that iodine deficiency disease appears in people. The manifestations of iodine deficiency disease that I describe here are far worse than the hypothyroidism commonly found in the United States (see Chapter 5) because the hypothyroidism in these situations begins when babies are conceived. Their mothers were already hypothyroid. Unless and until the chain of iodine deficiency is broken by providing sufficient iodine, the disease will continue to disrupt the lives of a quarter of the world's population.

Endemic cretinism is the term used for the group of signs and symptoms that are found in severe iodine deficiency disease. The Pan American Health Organization has defined endemic cretinism. It consists of several features:

✔ It's associated with endemic goiter and severe iodine deficiency. *Endemic goiter* means that more than 5 percent of children age 6 to 12 have enlarged thyroid glands.

✓ Patients are mentally deficient and also show either

• predominantly nervous system symptoms (like defects of hearing and speech) as well as defects when they stand and walk, called *nervous cretinism,* or

• symptoms of hypothyroidism and stunted growth called *myxedematous cretinism*

✓ Where iodine has been adequately replaced, cretinism does not occur.

Figure 12-1 shows a typical goiter on a person living in an area of endemic cretinism.

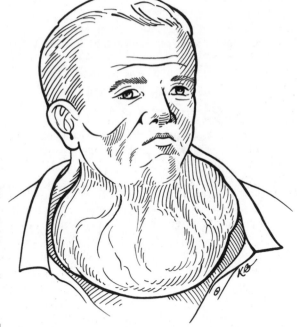

Figure 12-1:
A typical goiter for a person living in an area of endemic cretinism.

Looking at the geographic distribution

Endemic cretinism is found in the mountain regions of the world, as I explain earlier in the chapter. It's most common in the Andes and the Himalayas. It was found in the Alps until iodine replacement began several decades ago, but there are still areas in the Alps where people do not get sufficient iodine. It's found in mountainous regions of China, the Pacific, and the Middle East. It's also found in lowlands away from the ocean where heavy rains wash iodine out of the soil. It's present in central Africa, in central Brazil, and even in Holland.

In Europe, iodine deficiency disease remains a significant problem in numerous countries, including Austria, Belgium, Bulgaria, the Commonwealth of Independent States (including Russia), Croatia, Germany, Greece, Holland, Hungary, Ireland, Portugal, Romania, Spain, and Turkey.

Australia has this problem in its mountainous regions, especially Tasmania.

In South Asia, iodine deficiency disease is common in Bangladesh, India, Nepal, Tibet, and Pakistan.

In Southeast Asia, large populations of people with goiters are found in Burma, Vietnam, Thailand, and New Guinea.

In Latin and South America, large populations lack iodine in Bolivia, Brazil, Chile, Ecuador, Mexico, Peru, and Venezuela — mostly in the Andes Mountains and the mountains of Mexico.

In Africa, endemic cretinism is found in Cameroon, the Central African Republic, Nigeria, Uganda, Rwanda, the Sudan, Tanzania, Zaire, and Zimbabwe.

Contributing factors

Lack of iodine is, without a doubt, the main factor in endemic cretinism, but other issues definitely play a role in different areas of the world. Dietary factors other than iodine consumption are a major aspect of iodine deficiency disease.

In some areas of iodine deficiency disease, the normal diet includes substances that are harmful to the thyroid. In Africa, for example, cassava is a major part of the diet. Cassava contains cyanide, which is destroyed only if the food is properly prepared. If not, the cyanide is converted to thiocyanate in the body. Thiocyanate competes with iodine for uptake by the thyroid, thus decreasing even further the tiny amount of iodine that gets into the thyroid. (If someone consumes sufficient iodine, it overcomes any block from thiocyanate.)

Soybeans also interfere with thyroid function, preventing the production of thyroid hormone in the thyroid gland (see Chapter 10). Again, sufficient iodine can overcome the block and permit normal production of thyroid hormone, but when iodine is scarce, this extra loss of thyroid hormone can make a huge difference.

A third group of foods that may contribute to endemic cretinism is the Brassica group of vegetables, which includes foods such as broccoli and cauliflower. Hypothyroidism is more common in areas where these vegetables make up a large part of the diet and the diet is deficient in iodine.

Other foods that impair thyroid hormone production and are significant sources of food calories in certain areas of the world are bamboo shoots, sweet potatoes, corn, and lima beans.

Another important contributing factor in the development of iodine deficiency disease is the absence of selenium in the diet in certain areas, especially in China, Siberia, Korea, Tibet, and Central Africa. These are places where iodine deficiency is already present. *Selenium* is a mineral that the body needs in order to create the enzyme that turns T4 into the more potent T3.

Selenium may play a role in reducing the number of goiters associated with iodine deficiency. The enzyme in the thyroid that selenium helps to produce also has the function of disposing of hydrogen peroxide, a side product of thyroid hormone production. A buildup of hydrogen peroxide may destroy thyroid cells, leading to a small thyroid. But the small thyroid is still not healthy, despite the lack of a goiter.

When both selenium and iodine are absent from the diet, a disease called *Kashin–Beck disease* develops. This disease can lead to short stature as a result of the destruction of the growth-plates of bones, the *cartilage*. The damage is different than that seen in the short stature associated with myxedematous cretinism, which I describe later in the chapter. Kashin–Beck disease was previously thought to result from selenium deficiency alone, but it seems that the combination of deficiencies makes the disease even worse.

Goiter: The body's defense

The thyroid and the rest of the body do what they can to prevent hypothyroidism. The first response is a fall in the production of T4. When this drop occurs, the pituitary gland does not sense sufficient T3 in the brain, and it responds by secreting more TSH (see Chapter 3). The thyroid reacts by getting larger, thus forming a goiter, and by making more of the active hormone T3 (relative to the amount of T4). At the same time, the body converts more T4 into T3 away from the thyroid.

If the intake of iodine is severely limited, T3 production starts to fall. The consequence is severe hypothyroidism, which is particularly damaging in the brain.

Neurologic cretinism

It is believed that neurologic cretinism results from a lack of thyroid hormone from the mother during the period of the third to the sixth month of pregnancy. The severe iodine lack means that the growing fetus is unable to contribute thyroid hormone either. During this time period, the brain should be achieving the ability to hear as well as perform important motor functions, so those are the abilities most affected in this form of cretinism.

Neurologic cretinism has three major characteristics:

- Mental deficiency or retardation, although memory and social functions are unaffected

- Deafness and often loss of speech

- Stiffness of the arms and legs and an increase in the reflexes (opposite to what would be expected in hypothyroidism). The result is that this individual has a shuffling gait or may not be able to walk at all.

Neurologic cretins may not be hypothyroid later in life. If they receive sufficient iodine, they can have a thyroid that makes sufficient thyroid hormone. But the damage done by the lack of thyroid hormone during development of the brain cannot be undone.

Myxedematous cretinism

People with myxedematous cretinism are not as mentally retarded as those with neurologic cretinism. They don't tend to be deaf or mute as a result of their cretinism. Instead, they demonstrate the signs and symptoms of severe hypothyroidism from birth, including:

- Very dry, scaly, and thickened skin

- Retarded growth

- Thin hair, eyelashes, and eyebrows

- Puffy features

- Delayed sexual maturation

People with this condition do not have enlarged thyroids, but their thyroids are often replaced by scar tissue. As a result, their uptake of radioactive iodine is reduced despite having very high TSH levels. The levels of T4 and T3 hormones are very low. Many individuals have a combination of these two conditions.

Just why there should be such a difference between the two conditions is not clear. It may have to do with social forces in various cultures. In the Andes, where neurological cretins are more often found, there is a tradition of taking extraordinary care of these very handicapped individuals. This tradition of caring may not be present in places where such cretins are not often found. In those places they have not received the kind of care required and therefore have died. Or the environment may be too severe for the neurological cretin to survive in some areas but not in others.

A study done by Dr. Stephen Boyages and published in the *Journal of Clinical Endocrinology and Metabolism* in 1988 sheds some light on this subject. He studied a group of cretins in Qinghai Province in China and found both neurological and myxedematous cretins along with a mixed group. The difference between the types of cretins could be explained by the length of time that they were hypothyroid after birth, the myxedematous cretins having suffered for a longer time than the neurologic cretins. The neurologic cretins, after suffering mental retardation from a lack of thyroid hormone during brain development, had become normal with respect to thyroid function by getting enough iodine for the production of normal amounts of thyroid hormone after being born. Myxedematous cretins had thyroid destruction, while neurologic cretins had normal thyroid function. The conclusion of the researchers was that these two disorders are actually the same, only modified by the amount of hypothyroidism after birth.

Managing the Problem of Iodine Deficiency

You may think that managing the problem of iodine deficiency disease — preventing all goiters, cretinism, thyroid-related retardation, and hypothyroidism — should be easy. The trick is just to get everyone to eat sufficient iodine. The daily requirement is less than a pinhead of iodine. Over the lifetime of an individual, only a teaspoon of iodine is required. But consuming enough iodine is much easier said than done. And sufficient iodine consumption must occur prior to the conception of a baby in order to prevent the occurrence of cretinism.

A sprinkle of salt

As far as food sources of iodine, the highest content is found in fish and, to a lesser extent, milk, eggs, and meat. Fruits and vegetables contain very little iodine. Using iodine-rich foods to solve the problem is not likely to be successful, though, because diets and tastes differ throughout the world, and the logistics of transporting sufficient daily amounts of fish, milk, eggs, or meat to everyone in the world are overwhelming.

Because virtually every culture in the world uses salt, which is cheap and simple to iodize, iodized salt has been the standard way of overcoming the problem of iodine deficiency disease. The amount of salt needed to carry the daily requirement of 200 to 300 micrograms of iodine is very small and easily consumed.

In many countries, salt iodization has worked well, but some of its success has been less than glowing. Numerous international meetings have set goals and dates by which those goals should be attained. Charitable organizations, particularly the Kiwanis Clubs, have made the elimination of iodine deficiency disease a major goal. In some areas this goal of elimination of iodine deficiency has been achieved, but in many other areas, the problem continues to exist.

One major organization, the International Council for the Control of Iodine Deficiency Disorders (ICCIDD), serves as the central organization for coordination of these efforts. This organization has created the *global iodized salt logo,* which is placed on packages of salt that have been properly iodized (see Figure 12-2).

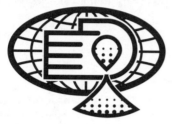

Figure 12-2:
The global
iodized salt
logo.

The history of efforts to overcome iodine deficiency disease in Bangladesh serves as an excellent illustration of the problems that are encountered. The UNICEF statistical summary for Bangladesh says that only 55 percent of households consume iodized salt, despite international efforts to rid the nation of iodine deficiency.

Bangladesh is subject to annual flooding with monsoon rains that have effectively washed all iodine out of the soil. The iodine has washed into the Bay of Bengal, which means that the fish caught there contain plenty of iodine. However, most of the population of the country lives in rural areas far from the supply of iodine. More than 50 million people in Bangladesh have goiters.

There has been a Law of Iodination in Bangladesh since 1984 that makes it illegal to sell salt in Bangladesh without iodizing it. However, no penalties were established until 1992. The cost of iodized salt in Bangladesh is 25 cents per kilogram, and non-iodized salt is 14 cents per kilogram. The poorest families buy the cheaper salt.

The cost of iodizing salt is only 5 cents per person per year. It's a simple process that can be done in a salt factory. But tests of iodine in salt show that as many as half the factories in Bangladesh are producing salt with insufficient iodine. In a country with a population the size of Bangladesh, this represents inadequate iodine intake for millions of people.

Some of the so-called iodized salt is not iodized at all in Bangladesh so that the provider can make an extra profit. Salt is sometimes brought in from other countries, mislabeled as iodized, and sold for a cheaper price than Bangladesh iodized salt. The country borders on Myanmar (formerly Burma) and India, which are not as strict in enforcing iodization. So smuggling contributes to iodine deficiency disease in Bangladesh as well.

One step in the right direction is the development of a simple kit by UNICEF that can detect whether salt contains iodine. A drop of liquid solution added to salt turns the salt blue if iodine is present. These kits are distributed to school children, who test their salt at home.

You can see that a successful iodization program involves much more than passing a law and setting up salt iodization programs in salt factories. A mountain of barriers can block such a simple solution.

An injection of oil

A highly effective way of managing iodine deficiency disorder is to inject iodized oil into the muscle of iodine deficient people. This substance is called *lipiodol,* and a single injection provides enough iodine to last for four years or longer. Lipiodol can also be taken by mouth, although it lasts only a little more than a year when consumed this way. Iodine given through this oil has resulted in significant shrinkage of goiters in just a few months. However, giving iodine injections also has its problems.

Iodine deficiency is found in rural areas where it's not always possible to give sterile injections. Qualified people are not always available to give the injections. Sufficient supplies of sterile needles and the iodized oil must be available. Also, in this age of AIDS, many people are reluctant to accept an injection. The oral form of lipiodol, of course, solves all these problems.

A slice of bread or cup of water

Other ways of managing iodine deficiency that have proven effective in some areas include the iodization of bread and the addition of iodine to the water supply. The problem with the iodization of bread is that bread consumption varies widely, and so this method works only in limited areas. Adding iodine to water doesn't work in areas with no public water supply, as is the case in most areas of the world where iodine deficiency disease is most prevalent.

Drawbacks of Iodization

One major problem that occurs when iodization programs are undertaken is the occurrence of hyperthyroidism when a lot of iodine is given to a person whose thyroid is under hyperstimulation with TSH. This happens with iodine injections and even with iodized salt that contains excessive iodine. The tools for managing hyperthyroidism (see Chapter 6) in a rural environment may not be readily available, especially if there are a large number of cases.

Chapter 13

Surgery of the Thyroid

. . . .

In This Chapter

▶ Determining whether you need surgery

▶ Picking the surgeon

▶ Preparing for surgery

▶ Understanding the procedure

▶ Managing after surgery

. . . .

*I*f you need to have a thyroid operation, the good news is that the thyroid is in a very convenient location. It's just a few millimeters under the skin of the neck, so it's easily found. Except in rare circumstances in which the gland is matted down and can't be freed up, thyroid surgery is not difficult in the hands of a skilled surgeon. Complications are few and infrequent, and the result of surgery is usually very satisfactory.

If you are about to have surgery, you need to know a few things to make the experience as benign as possible. Revealing those things is the purpose of this chapter. You probably won't be able to perform thyroid surgery after reading it (at least not after your first reading), but you will have a good idea of what to expect so that you won't get any surprises.

Deciding Surgery Is Necessary

Orlo Blunt is a 45-year-old man who has a solitary thyroid nodule — a lump on the thyroid. His doctor has performed a fine needle biopsy, which showed a *follicular lesion,* tissue that looks like normal thyroid follicles (the circles of cells that make thyroid hormone). The pathologist is uncertain whether the nodule is cancerous or not. Orlo is referred to Dr. Allen, a thyroid surgeon with extensive experience, for thyroid surgery. After examining Orlo, Dr. Allen tells him that he needs a *lobectomy* (the removal of one lobe of the thyroid). During the surgery, a pathologist will examine the tissue that has been removed. If the lobectomy shows that Orlo has follicular cancer, Dr. Allen will do a total *thyroidectomy* — he will remove the entire thyroid.

Orlo is sent for blood studies before the surgery, including thyroid function tests, which come back normal.

Orlo does not eat the morning of surgery. It is supposed to start at 7 a.m., but due to various glitches, the operation begins at 9 a.m. He is put under general anesthesia. The operation goes smoothly. The lesion proves to be a follicular *carcinoma* (cancer), so Dr. Allen performs a total thyroidectomy. Dr. Allen feels no nodes on the side of the thyroid but removes nodes in the central neck to look for cancer there. The pathologist determines that these nodes are not cancerous.

After the surgery, Orlo feels some soreness in his neck but is not hoarse. The incision on his neck is covered with a clear plastic bandage. Orlo has a chest X-ray and bone scan to make certain that cancer has not spread to those areas. These tests come back negative, indicating no cancer spread.

Several weeks after surgery, Orlo receives a dose of radioactive iodine (see Chapter 6) to destroy any remaining thyroid tissue. For the next several years, Orlo sees his doctor about every six months. The doctor finds no indications that the cancer is recurring.

He continues to be followed every six months for the next several years and does well with no evidence of recurrence.

A number of reasons might bring you to the thyroid surgeon. Orlo's situation is one of the most serious — thyroid cancer (see Chapter 8). But several other thyroid situations are best handled by surgery as well.

If you are hyperthyroid and antithyroid pills don't successfully treat your condition (or if you're allergic to them), and you don't want to have treatment with radioactive iodine, surgery is your only other choice. If you're pregnant and develop hyperthyroidism, and you're unable to take the antithyroid pills because of allergies, surgery is your only option. (You cannot be given radioactive iodine during pregnancy.)

If you have a large thyroid that is causing local symptoms in your neck, such as trouble swallowing or breathing, or if the goiter is especially unattractive, surgery is necessary, although radioactive iodine may be tried in these situations.

Finding Your Surgeon

The usual way that a surgeon is chosen is that your doctor picks your surgeon for you and you agree, assuming that he or she has your best interest at heart. In most cases, your doctor does have your best interest at heart, so this is a good method to follow. But sometimes other factors determine the doctor's choice as well. Perhaps the surgeon is an old friend and colleague with whom your doctor has been working for years. Or perhaps your doctor wants to keep your case within the confines of a particular hospital. (Occasionally, your insurance mandates that you can go only to certain surgeons.)

If your doctor does not choose your surgeon, your friend who has had surgery "somewhere in the neck area" or the lady behind the counter at the grocery store or the person who does your nails (assuming that you have them done) may have suggestions for surgeons. Personally, I wouldn't take this kind of recommendation when it comes to someone who is about to get under my skin.

The three most important criteria for a surgeon are experience, experience, and experience. If a surgeon does an operation once a month, that is not experience. If he or she does it several times a week, that's experience.

But how do you find a surgeon with the kind of experience you need? A number of organizations represent doctors who are particularly interested in thyroid surgery. The most important is the American Association of Endocrine Surgeons, which can be found on the Internet at www.endocrinesurgeons.org. At the site, you can click on "Search Our Membership Database" and choose a state. If you click on California, for example, you are presented with 23 names that I know include some of the best thyroid surgeons in the country. You can select your surgeon based upon his or her proximity to you, or you can go where the surgeon practices (assuming your insurance covers it).

Simply because a doctor is an endocrine surgeon does not mean that he or she specializes in thyroid surgery. There are many endocrine organs — the pancreas, the adrenals, the ovaries, and so forth — where the surgery is entirely different from thyroid surgery. Be sure you find a *thyroid* surgeon.

Another site that provides information about skilled thyroid surgeons is the site of the American Association of Clinical Endocrinologists at www.aace.com. Under "Services" you can "Find an Endocrinologist." From there you can select surgery as the specialty and choose the location. Another good resource is www.thyroid.org.

Don't go to a surgeon unless you're certain that you're ready for surgery. The job of the surgeon is to cut, and he or she probably won't try to talk you out of having surgery.

After you find a potential surgeon, your responsibility to your neck isn't over. You need to ask the surgeon some hard questions before you give him or her the privilege of cutting into you. The most important questions are the following:

> ✔ How often do you perform this surgery? (The answer should be more than three times a month, at least.)
>
> ✔ Have you had any deaths in the last five years while doing this surgery? (The answer had better be "no.")
>
> ✔ Have your patients had any serious and permanent complications from your surgery? (Keep reading in this chapter for information about specific complications.)

If you're happy with the surgeon's answers to these questions, go ahead and sign up.

Making Final Preparations Before Surgery

If you're having an operation for hyperthyroidism, you will probably take antithyroid pills for four to six weeks prior to surgery to get your thyroid function to be normal, which would be shown by a free T4 test. (If you can't take antithyroid pills because of an allergy, obviously you skip this step.) You often get iodine for ten days before surgery to reduce the size and blood vessels of the thyroid. You may also be placed on *propranolol,* a beta blocker, to control symptoms such as a rapid heartbeat or shakiness.

If you have hypothyroidism, you need to take thyroid hormone replacement pills prior to surgery so that your thyroid function is normal. Anesthesia is risky if a patient is very hypothyroid.

If you are taking aspirin or other medications like coumadin that thin the blood (and therefore prolong bleeding), you need to stop taking them a week before surgery.

A few days prior to surgery, you have blood tests to confirm that your organs such as your liver and kidneys are performing satisfactorily. The doctor also wants to confirm that you do not have anemia, although you won't lose much blood during thyroid surgery.

You should eat nothing after supper the night before surgery. The anxiety, the trauma of surgery, and the anesthesia all make you more prone to vomit, and you don't want to have anything in your stomach should this happen.

You generally come to the hospital on the morning of surgery. You are wheeled into the operating room, where the anesthesiologist gives you general anesthesia. (Sometimes you are given a local anesthesia, but this is unusual.) Two hours later, you awaken minus some or all of your thyroid. (It's not a great way to lose weight.)

What Happens During the Surgery

After all the preparations of cleaning and covering the area of the operation, the surgeon makes an incision about 3 inches long horizontally over the area of the thyroid. The surgeon can minimize the scar by carefully placing the incision over the normal skin fold (the place where your skin folds normally when you bend your head forward), and by making the smallest incision compatible with a given operation. If the surgeon has to remove lymph nodes, the incision may be carried up in the direction of the ear at one or both ends of the incision. The incision cuts through the fat underneath the skin and a thin muscle called the *platysma*. The skin and the muscle overlying the thyroid are pulled back to reveal the thyroid gland.

The surgeon then sees what he or she will be dealing with in the next hour or so. The thyroid is shaped like a butterfly, with an *isthmus* (a narrow strip) of thyroid tissue connecting the two "wings" of the butterfly. Above the isthmus, the surgeon may see a projection of thyroid tissue called the *pyramidal lobe*. This lobe is usually removed during any partial thyroid operation so that it will not regrow as a large bump on the front of the neck when the gland grows to restore thyroid hormone production.

The surgeon knows that the thyroid is firmly fixed to the trachea and larynx in back, so any operation has to free it up before the surgeon can remove the thyroid tissue. He or she sees two *superior thyroid arteries* entering the thyroid from above and two *inferior thyroid arteries* entering the thyroid from below. A fifth artery sometimes enters the thyroid in its central portion from below. These arteries may have to be tied and cut depending upon how much of the thyroid is to be removed.

The surgeon must also deal with the thyroid veins. The *middle thyroid veins* connect to the thyroid from the side. These must be tied and cut. The veins connecting to the top of the thyroid, called the *superior thyroid veins,* are also tied and cut if the plan is to remove the entire lobe.

Between three and six parathyroid glands, as well as the recurrent laryngeal nerves (one on each side), are found on the back of the thyroid and must be carefully preserved if possible. (See "Surgical obstacles," the next section, for details.)

Studies have shown that if a dye is injected into the thyroid, it goes to the chain of lymph nodes on the trachea behind the isthmus. The surgeon knows that this chain is where to look first for the spread of cancer.

At this point, the purpose of the surgery determines what is done next. If a hot nodule (see Chapter 7) is being removed, the surgeon locates any blood supply to it, cuts and ties off the blood supply, and removes the nodule. If hyperthyroidism is the reason for surgery, the surgeon performs a *subtotal thyroidectomy,* leaving a few grams of the part of the thyroid nearest the trachea to avoid damaging the parathyroid glands.

Surgical obstacles

In any thyroid surgery, the main obstacles to easy surgery are the parathyroid glands and the recurrent laryngeal nerves.

Parathyroid glands

The *parathyroid glands* sit on the back of the thyroid and share blood supply with it. There are usually four of these tiny glands, but there may be more or less, and they can be found in many locations.

The parathyroids are responsible for managing the calcium level in the blood. If they aren't functioning, the calcium level falls. A patient whose parathyroids are not functioning may experience tingling in her lips and numbness in her hands or feet. Sometimes the trauma of surgery causes the parathyroids to shut off temporarily, but they recover in a few days.

When a total thyroidectomy is done, preserving the parathyroid glands is often not possible. In that case, they are cut into small pieces and injected back into a muscle, for example in the shoulder, where they seem to function just fine.

If a patient has symptoms of low calcium after surgery, the problem can usually be managed with oral calcium supplements. Rarely, intravenous calcium is needed. If, by chance, the parathyroids do not recover their function after surgery, the patient takes vitamin D and calcium for life. This is a rare occurrence associated with only 1 in 300 surgeries of the thyroid.

Recurrent laryngeal nerves

The recurrent laryngeal nerves on both sides of the thyroid can be major obstacles to the surgeon. Each nerve controls the vocal cord on its side. Both nerves lie close to the thyroid and can easily be cut accidentally or included in a knot that is tying off a blood vessel. If the diagnosis is thyroid cancer, one or both of the recurrent laryngeal nerves may already be included in the cancer and have to be sacrificed at the time of surgery.

The recurrent laryngeal nerves may be temporarily damaged by the trauma of surgery. If so, the patient has a hoarse voice for a few days after surgery. If both are damaged, the situation is more serious, and a tracheostomy may be needed so the patient can breathe. The damage and the hoarseness may be permanent.

Damage to a recurrent laryngeal nerve should be very rare. In good hands, it doesn't happen more often than once for every 250 operations on the thyroid.

The superior laryngeal nerve may be injured during surgery as well. Damage to this nerve produces milder symptoms than those of recurrent laryngeal loss. Loss of this nerve produces voice fatigue and a decrease in the range of the voice.

Extent of surgery

A debate rages about how much thyroid to remove when a cancer is present in the thyroid. Most of the debate concerns small thyroid cancers — those that measure less than 1.5 centimeters in diameter. It seems that the survival rate for this size cancer is just as good whether a total thyroidectomy or less than a total thyroidectomy is done. Less than a total thyroidectomy would leave thyroid tissue in the area of the recurrent laryngeal nerve in order to avoid damaging it.

A *total thyroidectomy* is an attempt to remove all visible thyroid tissue. It's an extensive surgery that is more difficult than partial removal of the thyroid. A total thyroidectomy results in more frequent damage to parathyroids and nerves. Therefore, many surgeons do a *subtotal thyroidectomy,* leaving a small piece of one lobe of the thyroid intact, when the tumor is this small.

Other surgeons elect to do a total thyroidectomy on all thyroid cancer patients. They offer fairly convincing arguments:

- The morbidity and mortality rate of this surgery in their hands is very low.

- Thyroid cancer is often *bilateral,* meaning that it affects both lobes of the thyroid. If radiation is the cause of cancer, it's almost always bilateral.

- Scanning for evidence of new tumors, and treating any new tumors, is made much easier when no thyroid gland remains to take up radioactive iodine.

- After surgery, levels of thyroglobulin in the blood fall to zero. Therefore, if blood tests later show that a patient's thyroglobulin levels are rising, that is a strong indicator that a tumor is recurring.

After all or part of the thyroid has been removed, the question arises as to whether to remove lymph nodes, especially if none are enlarged. Many surgeons remove nodes over the trachea because cancer often spreads there first. They biopsy nodes to the side of the thyroid if they're enlarged, and they remove most of those nodes if the tissue has cancer. This is called a *modified radical neck dissection.* A more extensive form of this surgery is called an *unmodified radical neck dissection,* which involves removing muscles and other tissues. No study has ever shown that mortality is improved by this extensive surgery; it leaves the patient disfigured for no reason.

The surgeon attempts to remove as much cancer and thyroid as possible if the tumor is the undifferentiated type (see Chapter 8). By the time surgery is performed, these tumors usually have already spread, and little can be done. But surgery can help slow the inevitable local spread of this aggressive type of tumor.

A tumor of the medullary type (see Chapter 8) is managed with a total thyroidectomy and the removal of the central nodes around the trachea; lateral nodes to the side of the thyroid are removed only if they are visibly enlarged. Medullary tumors often secrete hormones that cause diarrhea or stimulate the adrenal gland, so removing as much tissue as possible prevents or reverses these complications.

If a surgeon has any concern about bleeding after surgery, or if so much tissue has been removed that a large space is left in the neck, the surgeon leaves a drain in the wound. A drain is needed only rarely and is usually removed after a day or two in any case. The drain helps prevent fluid accumulation and results in a better cosmetic outcome.

Considering a New Approach

Recently, surgeons have been trying a less invasive approach to thyroid surgery called *endoscopic thyroid surgery*. This is done when a diagnosis of cancer is uncertain and a nodule needs to be removed. A tiny tube is inserted in the neck, and a stream of carbon dioxide gas opens up the area. The surgeon uses high magnification to see the area in excellent anatomical detail. Another tube inserted into the area has a cutting edge that allows for removal of the nodule. The result is a less unsightly scar and a quicker return to activity for most patients, although the amount of pain that these patients feel is about the same as those who have a conventional operation.

This surgery may take a little longer than an open operation. If cancer is found during the endoscopic surgery, the surgeon usually opens the neck to proceed with an open, total thyroidectomy. However, this operation is promising as a way to avoid large scars and shorten the time between surgery and returning to work. As surgeons gain more experience with this method, it may start to replace the open operation.

Recuperating After the Operation

Earlier in the chapter, I note what occurs if you suffer recurrent laryngeal nerve damage or the loss of parathyroid gland function. You need to know about a few other possible complications from thyroid surgery. They are rare, but they do occur.

One complication is bleeding. If it's going to occur, it happens in the first few hours after surgery and occasionally requires that the surgeon go back and tie off the bleeding vessels. There's often some bandage placed over the site of the operation. If the bandage is too tight and bleeding occurs, the bleeding can compress the trachea and cause breathing difficulties.

Any surgery opens up the possibility of wound infection, which responds to antibiotics.

Any patient who has had extensive removal of the thyroid needs to take thyroid hormone replacement for life. If the operation is for thyroid cancer, you are given enough thyroid hormone to mildly suppress your thyroid-stimulating hormone (TSH).

Most people leave the hospital the same day of the surgery if none of these complications develop, which is usually the case.

It usually takes about a week to recover from the surgery. During that time, you feel some neck stiffness and tenderness. Your throat is sore and your voice is hoarse. You have a cough for a few days and feel some pain when you swallow. The scar becomes hard initially and then softens over the next month. An occasional patient forms a very thick scar called a *keloid*. This will be permanent since attempts to remove a keloid with plastic surgery often result in new keloid formation.

The only postoperative restriction is that you should not submerge in water for the first day or two. You can drive a car as soon as your head can turn without difficulty. Many people are back at work in two weeks. The surgeon often wants to see you again about three weeks after surgery to check on your results.

Chapter 14

The Genetic Link to Thyroid Disease

*I*n Chapters 2, 5, and 6, I introduce you to several members of the Dummy family: Sarah, Margaret, Stacy, Karen, and Tami. The reason these five women all come from the same prestigious family is that thyroid diseases often run in families. Many (though not all) thyroid diseases are inherited.

In this chapter, I discuss the various thyroid diseases that are inherited and how they are passed from one generation to the next. The progress that has been made in the last decade alone in understanding the inheritance of thyroid disease is nothing short of amazing. But all this new information has made the subject pretty complicated.

I try to clear up some of the complications in this chapter, but I'll be honest: This subject is not for the faint-hearted. If you're interested in knowing how your body is programmed to experience a certain disease, this chapter will definitely tickle your intellect. If you're reading this book solely to determine how to treat your present thyroid condition, you may want to head over to that chapter instead.

Even if the term *genetics* strikes fear in your heart, you may want to jump to the end of the chapter (the section called "The Future of Managing Hereditary Thyroid Disease") to discover some of the exciting ways that scientists are attempting to prevent thyroid and many other genetic diseases from being inherited in the future.

Genetics 101

To understand how the thyroid is affected by genetic disease, you need a basic understanding of genetics. This section provides the background that you need. This is not a book about genetics, so I've made this section as brief as possible while still giving you the essentials.

A monk and his pea plants

Although he never got credit for it in his lifetime, Gregor Mendel, an Austrian monk, is the starting point for all the great discoveries in *genetics,* the science of heredity. Mendel studied pea plants, looking at the ways that various characteristics of the plants were inherited, such as height, whether the seed was smooth or wrinkled, whether the pods were plump or pinched, and so forth.

Mendel knew that pea plants form new seeds when the pollen (which functions the same as sperm) in the male part of the plant called the *anther* (which is not quite the same as the penis) manages to attach to the *stigma,* the female part (not quite the same as the vagina), and get down to the ovary (the egg), which it fertilizes. The result is a seed, which grows into a plant.

Mendel carefully controlled the fertilization of his pea plants so that he knew which plant provided the pollen and which plant provided the ovary. He took, for example, the pollen of short pea plants that had never produced anything but short pea plants, and used it to fertilize the ovaries of tall pea plants that had never produced anything but tall pea plants. Then he took the pollen from tall pea plants and fertilized the ovaries of short pea plants. The result in both cases was always tall pea plants.

Mendel then crossed the tall offspring from this first fertilization (called the *first cross*) with each other. The offspring of the second cross were not all tall: Three-fourths were tall, and one-fourth was short. When Mendel crossed the short plants from the second cross with other short plants from the second cross, the result was plants that were always short. But if he crossed the short ones with the tall plants from the second cross, the new plants were usually, but not always, tall. The same pattern held true for the other characteristics that Mendel studied.

On the basis of these studies, Mendel made the following observations in the pea plant:

- A feature of the pollen and the egg determines whether a plant is tall or short. (This feature is now called a *gene;* Mendel did not use this term.)

- When the gene from the tall plant combines with the gene from the short plant, they do not mix to form an average plant.

- If a plant has two characteristics for the same gene such as tallness and shortness, one tends to be found more often than the other when they are crossed. (The gene that produces the trait found more often is the *dominant* gene, and the gene producing the trait found less often is the *recessive* gene.)

- There can be two different genes for a trait. (Two genes that determine the same trait are called *alleles*.)

- When plants are crossed that have two different traits, such as height and texture of the seed, these traits are passed to the offspring independently of one another. For example, a tall plant is not always found with a smooth seed or always with a wrinkled seed. Mendel concluded that genes (what he called *atoms of inheritance*) follow the principle of *independent assortment:* Each trait is inherited separately from all other traits.

Mendel's work received little attention when it was announced in 1865, but it was rediscovered in 1900. He got posthumous credit for his discoveries (for what that was worth).

Talk the talk

Using Mendel's research, scientists began to create the new language of genetics so that you and I could not possibly understand what they were talking about. I'm going to test my interpretation skills here to walk you through the maze they have created.

First, if a person (or a plant, dog, or chimpanzee) has two copies of the same allele, he or she is said to be *homozygous* for that gene. If he or she has one of each allele, the person is *heterozygous* for that gene. (We now know that, within a population, there can be more than two different alleles for each gene. However, any given person, animal, or plant has only two alleles for each gene.)

The appearance of the trait controlled by a gene is called the *phenotype*, while the genes that make up that phenotype are called the *genotype*. For instance, two tall pea plants may have the same appearance (phenotype), while their genotype may be different. One plant may have only tall genes and is tall, while the other has a tall gene and a short gene and is still tall (because tallness is the dominant gene).

A quick quiz: Based upon your in-depth knowledge of genetics, can two short pea plants have different genotypes? The answer is no, because shortness is the recessive gene. If a tallness gene is thrown into the mix, the plant is tall. Therefore, all short pea plants must have only the genes for shortness.

The great divide

At the same time that the world was ignoring Mendel's work, great things were happening under the microscope. Scientists were seeing that tissues are made up of cells and that new cells come from the division of old cells. As two new cells form, the old cell produces two copies of everything so that each new cell has exactly what the old cell had.

One particular area of the cell, which looks like a cell within the cell, was especially intriguing to scientists. This area is called the *nucleus* of the cell. As two new cells are being formed, some substances in the nucleus double and separate so that each new cell gets a complete set of these substances, which are called *chromosomes*.

Over the years, scientists discovered that each plant and animal has a set of chromosomes, but the numbers of chromosomes may differ between species. For instance, humans have 23 pairs or 46 chromosomes, while chimpanzees have 24 pairs or 48 chromosomes. (But chimpanzee chromosomes look more like human chromosomes than ape chromosomes, so don't be thinking that you're so smart.) The whole process by which one cell becomes two is called *mitosis*.

Examining the division of egg cells and sperm cells (the so-called *germ cells*), scientists discovered that each of these cells contains only half the normal number of chromosomes. In humans, for example, each egg cell and each sperm cell has one set of 23 chromosomes (while other human cells have 46 chromosomes). When these cells divide to form more sperm or egg cells (through a process called *meiosis*), the result is again 23 chromosomes per cell. When the egg and the sperm join together in fertilization, the combination, called a *zygote,* has the normal number of 46 chromosomes.

When a zygote is formed, one set of its chromosomes comes from the female and one set of chromosomes comes from the male. When these chromosomes are examined in the zygote cell, they pair up two-by-two. The members of each chromosome pair are called *homologous* chromosomes.

As is always the case, there's an exception to this rule. But like the French say, *vive le difference.* Loosely translated, that means "thank goodness for this particular set of chromosomes." The set I refer to are the sex chromosomes that determine whether you are a boy or a girl. All other pairs of chromosomes have matched genes so that if there's a gene for a given characteristic on one of the chromosomes of the pair, the other chromosome will have a gene for that characteristic. While a female has two matched sex chromosomes (called *X chromosomes*), a male has two different sex chromosomes (called an *X chromosome* and a *Y chromosome*).

Genes, chromosomes, and the traits they create

You may be thinking, "Two genes for every trait, two sets of chromosomes . . . genes and chromosomes must be the same." The problem is that any given plant, animal, or human has far more traits than the number of chromosomes that they have. Recognizing this, scientists realized that chromosomes contain many genes, not one.

Genes for various traits are found on a single chromosome. Each chromosome is passed down to its *daughter cells* — the cells created when a cell divides. Therefore, some genes (and the traits they create) get passed down together from generation to generation. (They don't follow the principle of independent assortment.) Genes on the same chromosome are said to be *linked*.

Even though some genes are linked, they sometimes do get inherited independently, just as Mendel predicted. This happens because *crossing over* takes place. What is crossing over? During the process of meiosis, which produces sperm and egg cells, as the sets of chromosomes line up close together, genes on one chromosome can cross over to the other while their alleles cross over in the other direction. In this way, *recombinant* chromosomes are formed — new combinations that help to make your offspring different from you.

The discovery of crossing over meant that chromosomes could start to be *mapped*. That is, scientists could determine which genes are on which chromosomes and where, because the closer two genes are, the less likely they are separated by a cross-over, while the further they are from one another, the more likely they are to separate.

Another way that a new trait replaces an old one is when a *mutation* takes place. As a result of faulty copying of the chromosome or an outside influence such as radiation, chemicals, or the sun, a new gene replaces an old one. Usually mutation isn't noticed, either because the gene is recessive or because the mutation may kill the individual so that it isn't reproduced. Once in a while, a mutation is good for the animal or plant in which it occurs, producing a useful trait.

The secret lives of genes

Genes are made up of long, long, long chains of *nucleic acids.* Nucleic acids have three components: a sugar called *deoxyribose;* a *phosphate* attached at one end of the sugar; and a *base,* which may be adenine, cytosine, guanine, or thymine, attached to the sugar at another point. The genes are said to contain *deoxyribonucleic acid* or DNA.

Within the DNA, the number of adenine molecules is always equal to the number of thymine molecules, while the cytosine equals the guanine. In 1952, biochemists James D. Watson and Francis H. C. Crick showed that this equality is because each gene contains two chains of nucleic acids. The adenine on one chain is always paired with the thymine on the other, while cytosine on one chain is always paired with guanine on the other. Other researchers had shown that DNA has a helical structure, so Watson and Crick called the structure a *double helix* — a shape that looks like a spiral staircase.

One of the best things about the identification of the double helix was that it became clear how the genes could copy themselves or *replicate:* The helix could break apart into two strands. The two individual strands then each act as a template so that a new strand forms on each in the only way it can, by connecting to the only nucleic acid it can combine with — namely, a nucleic acid containing adenine connects to a nucleic acid containing thymine, and a nucleic acid containing cytosine connects with a nucleic acid containing guanine. The result is two new double helixes.

Next, the DNA has to somehow control the creation of the animal or plant and the ongoing processes that allow it to live. It does so by producing *ribonucleic acid,* or RNA. RNA is made up of nucleic acids just like DNA, but the sugar in RNA is ribose and the bases are adenine, cytosine, and guanine, with uricil replacing thymine.

In the same way that the double helix can break apart to reproduce itself, it can break apart and construct a complementary RNA molecule. This process is called *transcription.* The RNA remains a single strand, not a double helix. It's called *messenger RNA* because it serves to carry the message from the DNA to the next level of control, the enzyme. An *enzyme* is a protein that acts as a facilitator for a chemical reaction — for example, the breakdown of a complex carbohydrate like glycogen (the storage form of glucose — the body's source of immediate energy) into small glucose molecules that can be instantly used.

The messenger RNA accomplishes its task by acting as a template in its turn for the production of the enzyme or protein. This process is called *translation.* Proteins are made up of amino acids. Every three bases in the messenger RNA, called a *triplet,* causes one particular amino acid to line up opposite them. Each group of three is a *codon,* because it codes for a specific amino acid. By making up artificial messenger RNA that contained the same codon again and again, it was possible to determine which amino acid was selected by each codon.

With four different bases in sets of three, the maximum number of codons is 64, but there are only 20 amino acids. It was discovered that different codons select the same amino acid, and some codons act as the code for the end of a protein without selecting an amino acid.

Just to complicate things a little further, the amino acids don't actually line up opposite the codons but are carried at one end of another RNA molecule called *transfer RNA*. At its other end, transfer RNA has the bases that are complementary to the codon. So the transfer RNA lines up neatly against the messenger RNA, while the amino acids are lined up next to one another at the other end. A series of other steps that you don't need to know to understand hereditary thyroid disease then bind the amino acids into a protein that may be an enzyme or a muscle or whatever.

In higher animals, genes also contain large segments of bases that do not code anything and, in fact, have to be cut out from their complementary RNA before the RNA can produce a protein. These sequences are called *introns,* and their function is not known.

Shall I be a liver or a brain?

I show you earlier in the chapter that a fertilized egg reproduces itself by the process of mitosis, creating two identical cells. How can each identical cell transform itself into a thyroid cell or a liver cell or even a brain cell?

The gene utilizes a number of techniques to turn gene action on and off. There are short sequences of bases prior to the active gene called *promoters*. When various factors bind to a promoter, it turns on the action of the gene to begin transcription. Other sequences of elements called *enhancers* increase the activity of the gene further, while *silencers* tend to shut down the activity of the gene. The process of transcription from DNA to messenger RNA comes to a halt when certain sequences of bases are reached.

Because all cells contain the same genetic information, a thyroid cell differs from a brain cell as a result of the particular genes that are *expressed* (active) in each cell. Many different factors determine whether a gene is expressed or not. Promoters and enhancers increase their activity in response to various hormones or growth factors that may be present in one cell but not another.

The expression of a gene may be controlled at the level of the gene itself, or it may be controlled after transcription has taken place so that the messenger RNA never makes the protein.

In these and in many other ways yet to be discovered, cells utilize only the genes they need to function within their environment.

The Origins of Genetic Thyroid Diseases

Now that you have a basic understanding of genetics, you can apply your knowledge to thyroid diseases that are transmitted through inheritance. A child inherits a thyroid disease in one of three basic ways:

✔ A single gene from a parent may transmit a dominant or recessive trait to the child. This method goes back to Mendel and his peas.

✔ Many genes may be involved in the inheritance of a disease so that the child has to inherit all of them to get the disease.

✔ An entire chromosome may be abnormal, resulting in disease. For example, if a female ends up with only one X chromosome, that lack can produce a condition known as *Turner's syndrome,* which often includes a thyroid disorder.

Inheriting a disease through a single gene

Many diseases are inherited through a single gene, often as a result of a gene mutation. A disease may be inherited as a recessive gene, which means that both parents must supply the same gene in order for the disease to appear. It may be inherited as a dominant gene, so that only one parent supplies the gene necessary to cause the disease. Or a disease may be inherited with the X chromosome in a recessive form, which means that a male will get the disease (because he has only one X chromosome), but a female is spared unless both her X chromosomes have the gene.

The entire list of diseases transmitted by single-gene inheritance may be found at www.ncbi.nlm.nih.gov/omim, the homepage of Online Mendelian Inheritance in Man (OMIM), a huge database compiled by Dr. Victor McKusick at Johns Hopkins University. If you search the term "thyroid" from the homepage, 344 different thyroid diseases are listed at the time of this writing. Each one is fully described, with citations of all the research that has been done to define the defect and a complete bibliography at the end of each description.

Recessive inheritance

Many conditions where thyroid hormone is not made properly fall into the category of recessive inheritance. It takes two "bad" genes to develop one of these conditions. If you have just one bad gene, you're a carrier of the disease, but you don't experience it yourself. The *phenotype* (the way this gene makes itself known) is usually a large thyroid that does not produce sufficient thyroid hormone. Note that several of the conditions appear to be the same because the final result of the condition is absence of thyroid hormone, but each condition involves a defect in a different step in the production of thyroid hormone. Among the conditions inherited this way are:

✔ **A defect in the production of thyroid hormone** (see Chapter 3): Patients with this condition are hypothyroid (see Chapter 5) and have goiters. This condition stems from an abnormality in the creation of the enzyme that produces thyroid hormone.

- **Thyroid hormone unresponsiveness:** If you inherit a bad gene instead of the gene that makes the receptor protein for thyroid hormone, your end organs are not responsive to the thyroid hormone your body produces. This condition causes patients to be deaf and have goiters. With this condition, the T3, T4, and TSH levels are all elevated (see Chapter 4).

- **Pendred Syndrome:** Patients with this disease are deaf and have goiters, but their thyroid function is normal. The disease also causes mental retardation and an increased tendency to develop thyroid cancer. The defect is in the production of thyroid hormone, but at some point it improves so that hypothyroidism is not present later on.

- **Thyroid transcription factor defect:** The patient has a goiter and decreased levels of thyroglobulin. If you remember that *transcription* is the term for the production of messenger RNA from DNA, you will understand where this defect arises.

- **Defect in thyroid production:** This is different from thyroid transcription factor defect. The patient is hypothyroid, has a goiter, and experiences mental retardation. Lab tests show a defect in the formation of thyroid hormone. Normally, two molecules of tyrosine with iodine attached couple together to form thyroid hormone, but this process fails in this particular inherited condition.

Dominant inheritance

Many inherited thyroid conditions are passed from parents to children this way: One "bad" gene produces the disease. These diseases tend to be more common than those inherited by recessive genes. Examples of diseases inherited this way are:

- **A thyroid hormone receptor defect:** If you have this condition, your body is resistant to the action of thyroid hormones. At the same time, you experience mild hyperthyroidism. Patients with this condition have short stature, learning disabilities, deafness, and goiters. Lab tests show high levels of T3, T4, and TSH.

- **Papillary thyroid carcinoma** (see Chapter 8). This type of cancer usually occurs at an earlier age than thyroid cancer that is not inherited.

- **A different defect in thyroid hormone receptor:** This produces a child with severe cretinism of the neurologic form (see Chapter 12).

- **Thyroid hormone resistance** (also found in a recessive form). A patient with this condition has a goiter and the child begins to speak at a later than expected age, but his thyroid function is normal. Lab tests show that T3 and T4 levels are high, but the TSH level is normal.

- **Multiple Endocrine Neoplasia, Type II:** This condition causes tumors on multiple organs, including medullary carcinoma of the thyroid (see Chapter 8), a tumor of another gland called the adrenal gland, and tumors of the parathyroid glands. Lab tests show increased levels of epinephrine and calcitonin in the blood.

✏ **Medullary Carcinoma of the Thyroid, Familial:.** Patients with this condition have medullary cancer (see Chapter 8).

X-linked inheritance

X-linked inheritance presents fewer examples because men have only one X chromosome and women have two, compared to 44 other chromosomes that can produce a disease by recessive or dominant inheritance. If a disease passed on by the X chromosome is recessive, both parents must give the gene to a daughter in order for the disease to appear, but a son gets the disease if only one parent passes along the gene. Some examples of diseases inherited this way include:

✏ **Immunodeficiency and Polyendocrinopathy:** A baby with this condition has unmanageable diarrhea, diabetes, and thyroid autoimmune disease. A child born with this condition usually dies very young.

✏ **Thyroid-binding globulin abnormality:** This condition produces retardation. Lab tests show that someone with this disease has decreased thyroid-binding globulin (see Chapter 3).

✏ **Multinodular goiter:** The thyroid is larger and multinodular (see Chapter 9).

Inherited thyroid diseases can affect every step in thyroid hormone production, transportation, and action. The ones I list here are only 14 of the 344 currently listed in the OMIM database. New conditions are being discovered all the time.

Inheriting a disease through multiple genes

The major thyroid disease that is inherited as a result of abnormalities of multiple genes is *autoimmune thyroiditis*. This disease is much more common in women than men, so you may assume that the inheritance is linked to the X chromosome somehow. But if this is the case, the method by which the X chromosome passes the disease along is not known. One idea is that the female sex hormone influences the occurrence of this disease, but just how this may happen is not understood.

Autoimmune thyroiditis is easy to diagnose because lab tests show that a person has autoantibodies (see Chapter 5) that damage the thyroid. Many genes are involved in the production of autoantibodies. The substance (such as thyroid tissue) that provokes antibodies is called an *antigen*. The antigen is first broken into small pieces that are bound to cells by way of proteins called *major histocompatibility molecules*. This combination of cells and antigens leads to the activation of another cell called the *T cell*. The T cell helps yet another cell, the *B cell*, recognize the antigen and produce antibodies against it. Multiple genes are involved in all these steps.

The major histocompatibility region of the chromosomes is on the short arm of chromosome 6. It determines which antigens are found on white blood cells. These antigens are the human leukocyte antigens (HLA). The antigens can be identified chemically. In this way, it has been shown that in whites, HLA-B8 and HLA-DR3 are the antigens associated with Graves' disease (see Chapter 6), while in Koreans, the DR5 and DR8 are most common. In Japanese, the antigen most associated with Graves' disease is DR5, and in Chinese, it's DR9. All of this is important because doctors can test for these antigens in relatives of affected individuals. If the antigens are present, they are more likely to get the disease.

Another disease that is found more often in people with certain human leukocyte antigens is postpartum thyroiditis (see Chapter 11). In whites, the antigens are HLA DR3, DR4, or DR5, while in Chinese, it is DR9.

Inheriting a chromosome abnormality

During the creation of a zygote, as new cells are being formed, it's possible to have a mistake in the division of the chromosomes into the two new cells so that one cell ends up with an extra chromosome and the other ends up with one less chromosome. The most well known conditions associated with this kind of chromosome mistake are Turner's syndrome and Down's syndrome. Both conditions are associated with hypothyroidism, but Down's syndrome is also associated with hyperthyroidism on occasion.

Down's syndrome results when the new cells that are created have an extra chromosome — they have three copies of the 21st chromosome instead of two. This condition has a typical physical appearance with facial features that are recognized at birth. A child with Down's syndrome has palms that have a single crease, and her muscles lack tone. Reduced intelligence and other abnormalities are part of this syndrome.

Turner's syndrome results when an X chromosome is left behind, so that a female with a single sex chromosome is produced. The patient has distinctive facial features including low-set ears, folds of skin in the inner corner of the eye, and drooping eyelids. The patient also may have diabetes mellitus, cataracts, rheumatoid arthritis, and cardiac abnormalities in addition to chronic thyroiditis.

The Future of Managing Hereditary Thyroid Disease

Up to now, scientists haven't been successful in their attempts to remove a "bad" gene from a human and replace it with a healthy gene — a process known as *genetic engineering*. The problem is that they don't yet know how to deliver the new gene successfully. If scientists can determine how to do so, they can open the door to preventing diseases that are inherited through a single gene.

Genetic engineering

If a disease is caused by a recessive gene, replacing that gene with its dominant form in sufficient amounts should be enough to cure the condition. Usually in a recessive gene disorder, the disease occurs because that particular gene is not functioning at all, so providing even a small level of function may cure the condition.

The disorders that would most easily respond to genetic engineering are disorders of the blood system, because blood is easily removed. A new gene can be spliced into the cells and the blood reintroduced to the patient. The first trial of gene therapy, performed in 1990, was for a disorder that resulted in severe loss of immunity so that the patient was very susceptible to any infection, as well as a cancer. Scientists were able to introduce the necessary gene into the blood cells of the patient by connecting it to a virus, which infected the cells and added the gene to their DNA. The cells were then cultured to increase their number and reinserted. Unfortunately, the trial didn't work, probably because the efficiency of splicing the gene into the cells was low.

Other genetic disorders for which trials of gene therapy have taken place include *familial hypercholesterolemia,* where excessive production of cholesterol leads to early death by heart attack; *cystic fibrosis,* where lack of a certain gene leads to excessive production of a thick mucous in the lungs that results in chronic lung infection; and *Duchenne muscular dystrophy,* where severe muscle deterioration leads to the individual dying by the third decade of life. A trial of gene replacement in all three of these conditions has been unsuccessful.

Another novel way of managing diseases caused by defective genes is to find a gene that is active during fetal life (but becomes dormant later on) and could replace the activity of the defective gene, if it could be made to express itself. A prime candidate for this treatment would be sickle cell disease. In this disease, abnormal hemoglobin (hemoglobin is the chemical in red cells that carries oxygen to the tissues of the body) leads to the early loss of red blood cells, which become sickled (crescent-shaped) in appearance and can block blood flow to tissues, causing great pain. A gene active during fetal life produces fetal hemoglobin, which does not sickle. If this gene can be turned on during adult life, it would replace the defective hemoglobin made by the patient. Scientists are looking for the drug that may be able to turn this gene on.

Cancer treatment has seen a lot of activity in the area of gene therapy. One approach has been to insert a gene that increases the sensitivity of the cancer to a drug, or to insert a poison into cells that are then injected directly into the tumor. Another approach is to insert a gene that increases the activity of the patient's immune system. Finally, some tumors arise when the activity of tumor suppressors (chemicals in the body that suppress the growth of tumors) declines. The treatment attempted aims to restore tumor suppressor activity with a new gene that is inserted into blood cells. All these treatments have seen some success, but no one has yet been cured of cancer with gene therapy. So far none of the cancer therapy trials have targeted thyroid cancer.

Scientists are also attempting to increase a tumor's immune response by modifying the tumor so that it provokes body cells against it. This is done by inserting genes into the tumor that cause it to produce new antigens that the body can fight against. Tumors like malignant melanoma and colon cancer have been the target of this type of therapy. A similar technique involves inserting a gene directly into a tumor that activates a cancer-killing agent, which is subsequently injected. These techniques have led to some decrease in tumor size but, so far, no cures of cancer. Interestingly, the use of gene therapy is not limited to tumors that have been brought on by faulty genes but can be directed at any tumor, genetic or not.

The ethics of germline gene therapy

You can see that the range of techniques for using genetic engineering to cure disease is enormous. New methods of delivering healthy genes to replace disease-conferring genes are being discovered as you read this book. This approach would certainly be the most simple and successful way of treating the diseases provoked by inheritance of a single dominant gene. However, this type of treatment would cure only the particular individual, without affecting the transmission of the disease to his or her offspring. To eliminate the disease from future generations, the genetic engineering would have to take place in the sperm and/or the egg, the *germline* of the individual.

Germline gene therapy raises tremendous ethical questions. If we have the tools for eliminating the recessively inherited Pendred syndrome by replacing a Pendred gene with a normal gene, don't we also have the tools for changing skin color, height, or any other body characteristic in future generations?

So far, germline gene therapy has actually been successful in some animals, but has not been done on humans for several reasons:

✔ The methods used so far are very imprecise, so that the final product is uncertain, including the possible introduction of harmful genes.

✔ Many people fear that germline gene therapy may lead to germline enhancement, an attempt to produce a "superior" human being.

✔ It's uncertain that germline gene therapy is even needed, because a harmful recessive trait requires mating with another human with the same trait to express itself, while dominant traits are present in only half of a germline. It makes more sense to identify the sperm or egg with the normal gene and use that in fertilization, rather than trying to modify the sperm or egg with the abnormal gene. Genetic testing of the germline should be done if these diseases are to be eliminated.

An entire field of genetics concerns *ELSI,* the ethical, legal, and social implications of genetic science.

Clearly, genetics is the current frontier in medical science. It promises to prevent or cure many of the diseases that plague humans, including hereditary thyroid disease and nonhereditary tumors, but the road to that cure is filled with cracks and bumps that will result in a very uneven ride.

Part IV
Special Considerations in Thyroid Health

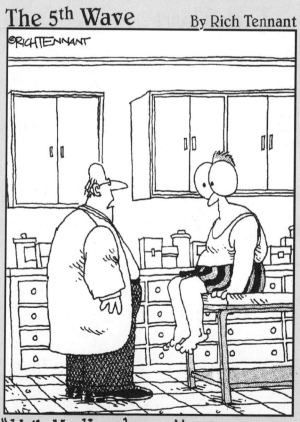

The 5th Wave   By Rich Tennant

"Well, Mr. Humphrey - it appears your thyroid isn't the only thing that's become enlarged."

In this part . . .

Certain groups are affected differently from the rest of us by thyroid disease. These include pregnant women, children, and elderly people. Their special needs are taken up in this part. Plus, there is plenty you can do to keep your thyroid happy and making those essential hormones in the right quantities. The last chapter in this part discusses some ways you can manage your body so that thyroid function takes place in a healthy environment.

Chapter 15

What's New in Thyroid Treatment?

I went online to a search page of the National Library of Medicine called "Pub Med" on April 18, 2001, and did a search for "thyroid disease." The result was 34,397 citations to studies that thousands of scientists have done in the last year or two that are published in medical journals. This research represents the cutting edge of medicine. But how do you stay on the cutting edge without slipping and getting sliced up? That's one of the reasons you bought this book: So I can do the work of sifting through that research for you.

In this chapter, you find a selection of the most important discoveries in thyroid medicine during the last couple years. Some are single studies of a subject that could be revised or even overturned when someone else does a similar study. You have to keep an open mind when new (and not necessarily validated) material such as this is presented.

As I write this chapter, new findings are being evaluated by scientific editors and getting ready to join the thousands of studies before them. It isn't possible to be up-to-the-minute in a book, given the constraints of a publishing deadline and the amount of information coming out. That's why I include Appendix B in this book — to point you toward Web site resources that can be updated more frequently than a book. Don't hesitate to make use of them.

Preventing Ill Effects of Large Doses of Iodine

Many of the agents that allow radiologists to view the insides of things, such as the bowels, contain a lot of iodine. Just how much does all this iodine affect thyroid function? That was what a group from Germany studied and published in the periodical *Endoscopy* in March 2001. They looked at 70 patients who didn't have thyroid disease. All had to have a test called — take a deep breath — an *endoscopic retrograde cholangiopancreatogram*. This study involved placing a tube into the bile duct system and injecting an iodine-containing agent to look for bile stones or other obstructions. Each patient got a large dose of iodine in the process. The thyroid glands of these patients were studied with an ultrasound examination (see Chapter 4) prior to their bile duct tests.

The researchers found that the iodine caused a lasting decrease in thyroid-stimulating hormone (TSH), especially in patients who had large thyroids with nodules. The free T3 hormone level increased in all patients, but the free T4 level increased particularly in the people who had enlarged nodular thyroid glands. The amount of iodine excreted in the patients' urine greatly increased after the test.

The conclusion of the study was that a thyroid ultrasound was the best way to evaluate patients for possible thyroid problems before giving them iodine-containing contrast agents.

If you need to have a test that requires you to receive a large dose of iodine, ask your doctor to check your thyroid carefully prior to the test. A thyroid ultrasound is probably the best test to rule out thyroid disease in this situation. The ultrasound can help you and your doctor prepare for the consequences of giving a lot of iodine to an abnormal thyroid gland.

Finding Out More about Hypothyroidism

Many recent studies focus on the proper treatment of hypothyroidism. The following sections offer just a sampling of the research that has been done in the last few years.

Treating (or not treating) subclinical hypothyroidism

One of the great debates in thyroid management is what to do about *subclinical hypothyroidism*. This is a condition where the patient's TSH level is slightly elevated (say to 6 or 7), the free T4 level is normal, and the patient has some nonspecific symptoms that could be the result of hypothyroidism or something else. Doctors have been studying these patients, looking for signs of low thyroid function or a response to thyroid medication, because they are not sure whether treatment is necessary or not.

One study from Italy, published in the *Journal of Clinical Endocrinology and Metabolism* in March 2001, looked at the function of the heart in 20 people with subclinical hypothyroidism, all of whom showed some abnormality in heart activity. Half of the study participants were given thyroid treatment, and the other half were given a placebo. The study found that people given the thyroid treatment drug showed an improvement in heart function, while those given a placebo showed no change. They concluded that people with subclinical hypothyroidism have measurable abnormalities that are improved with thyroid treatment.

Another study from Germany, published in *Thyroid* in August 2000, looked at heart disease and heart attacks in patients with subclinical hypothyroidism. The author found that these patients sustained a definite increase in heart disease and heart attacks over patients without the condition. Various tests of normal heart function, such as changes in heart rate with exercise, indicated that those functions were impaired in people with subclinical hypothyroidism. The most at-risk people were women over age 50 who smoked and had TSH levels greater than 10. Giving the study patients thyroid medication improved these functions and also improved the levels of fats in the blood. The author of this study felt that these changes justified the use of thyroid treatment in subclinical hypothyroidism. He noted, however, that giving a patient replacement thyroid hormone tends to speed up the heart rate and may worsen chest pain, which must be considered when treating someone with this condition.

If you have a diagnosis of subclinical hypothyroidism, you and your doctor should look carefully for subtle evidence of low thyroid function and treat the condition with replacement thyroid hormone if such evidence is found.

Finding the right dose of hormone

A question that keeps coming up among doctors who treat hypothyroidism is "What is the correct dose of thyroid medication?" Some physicians believe that lowering a patient's level of thyroid-stimulating hormone (TSH) to under 5 is sufficient to eliminate signs and symptoms of low thyroid function, but many patients are still symptomatic at that level. In a study published in the *Medical Journal of Australia* in February 2001, the authors show that lowering the TSH to between 0.3 and 2.0 may be beneficial. Furthermore, some

patients do much better when their thyroid hormone replacement pills
contain both types of thyroid hormone: T3 as well as T4. (Most pills that
patients currently take contain T4 replacement hormone only.)

If you are being treated for hypothyroidism and still have symptoms associated
with low thyroid function when your TSH level is between 3 and 5, ask your
doctor to treat you to lower that level. I believe that doing so will improve
your health.

Determining the prevalence of hypothyroidism

How common is thyroid disease in the population? A group in Norway
studied this question and published their answer in the *European Journal of
Endocrinology* in November 2000. They looked at the TSH levels of people
who supposedly had no thyroid disease and found that they were between
0.49 and 5.7 for females and 0.56 and 4.6 for males. If they then excluded the
patients who tested positive for thyroid autoantibodies, which indicates that
they may be prone to thyroid disease, the range of "normal" TSH numbers
dropped to 0.49 to 1.9 in the women. (The study did not report the range for
the men.) The conclusion these researchers arrived at is that despite a huge
number of recognized cases of thyroid disease in the population, a significant
number of cases are not recognized.

This study offers further proof that the correct normal range for TSH (a range
that excludes any person with thyroid disease) is lower than the one that is
quoted by most laboratories.

Linking depression to hypothyroidism

Hypothyroidism has been associated with depression (see Chapter 2). It is
very important to consider this link when treating depressed patients,
because treating the thyroid may cure the depression.

In a study in the *Annals of Pharmacotherapy* in October 2000, the authors
present a woman who had long-standing depression. Even when she took a
very large dose of T4 thyroid replacement hormone — up to 0.3 mg daily —
she continued to be depressed. However, when a low dose of T3 hormone
was added to the treatment, her mood improved significantly.

Based on the findings of this study, if you have hypothyroidism and are
depressed despite taking replacement T4 hormone, ask your doctor whether
replacement T3 hormone can be added to your treatment.

Heart disease and hypothyroidism

A study in *Thyroid* in1999 pointed out that *homocysteine,* a substance found in the blood, is an independent risk factor (like high blood pressure, smoking, and high cholesterol) for arteriosclerotic heart disease. Because heart disease is commonly found in patients with hypothyroidism, the authors of the study looked for levels of homocysteine in these patients. They found that levels were abnormally high in these patients, and the levels fell when patients took thyroid hormone replacement. The authors suggest that the combination of abnormal fats (especially cholesterol) and high levels of homocysteine may be the reason that hypothyroid patients are at risk for heart attacks.

Dealing with Hyperthyroidism

Despite the availability of several treatments for hyperthyroidism (see Chapter 6), specialists are not satisfied with any of them. Each treatment is associated with either frequent failure or undesirable side effects like hypothyroidism. The search for better therapy continues.

Measuring calcium levels

A new study published in January 2001 emphasizes the importance of measuring calcium levels of patients with thyroid conditions, especially hyperthyroidism. This German study shows that after thyroid surgery, *hypoparathyroidism* — the loss of parathyroid function — frequently occurs and leads to low calcium levels. (A high calcium, on the other hand, may be caused by *hyperparathyroidism* — excess parathyroid function. In this study, excess parathyroid function was also relatively common in association with thyroid disease.)

Harry, the hyperthyroid horse

Hyperthyroidism is managed in a variety of ways. However, for a horse named Harry, surgery was the only consideration. Harry's case was reported in the *Journal of the American Veterinary Medical Association* in October 2000. He suffered from all the symptoms that people show (see Chapter 6), including fever, nervousness, and weight loss. His thyroid was prominent, especially on the right side. Harry was treated with surgery to remove the overactive lobe and responded very well.

Both decreased and increased parathyroid function are found at a higher rate in patients with hyperthyroidism than in people who don't have thyroid disease. If you have hyperthyroidism, be sure to have your calcium level checked regularly.

Controlling weight gain

Many hyperthyroid patients are concerned about getting treatment because they fear that they'll gain weight when their thyroid function decreases.

In a study from Edinburgh, Scotland, published in the journal *Thyroid* in December 2000, the authors compared patients treated for hyperthyroidism who have become hypothyroid as a result of treatment. Their study shows that patients who started taking T4 thyroid hormone replacement immediately after their treatment (because they quickly became hypothyroid) gained much less weight than patients who delayed starting hormone replacement because their TSH levels were normal.

The authors concluded that defining hypothyroidism using the usual range of TSH after treatment of hyperthyroidism leads to many people not getting the treatment they need. It is well known that TSH levels tend to lag behind (remaining low) as the patient resumes normal thyroid function or even becomes hypothyroid after treatment of hyperthyroidism. In this situation, clinical symptoms and a reduced free T4 level are better indicators than the TSH level of the need for treatment.

Revolutionizing thyroid surgery

A new type of thyroid surgery being tested uses tiny scopes instead of an incision in the neck. This surgery has been tested for removing thyroid nodules. In a paper from Japan published in *Surgery Today* in 2001, the authors discuss the use of an "endoscopic" technique. Using carbon dioxide to raise the skin, the doctors were able to remove the thyroid successfully in 12 patients. One patient did have postoperative *hypoparathyroidism* (low parathyroid function) and recurrent laryngeal nerve injury (see Chapter 13). However, the results were very satisfactory for the patients, who experienced no scars and little blood loss. If this technique continues to show this degree of success as more patients are treated, it should become an option for most hyperthyroid patients in the next few years.

Gathering clues to hyperthyroid eye disease

Just exactly why hyperthyroid eye disease occurs is not clear, but researchers generally believe that it has a basis as an autoimmune disorder (see Chapter 4 for a discussion of thyroid autoantibodies). One suggestion is that thyroglobulin enters the muscles of the eyes, and antibodies react against it. A study from Italy in the journal *Thyroid* in 2001 showed that thyroglobulin could, indeed, be found in the muscle tissue of the eyes. The study demonstrated that the thyroglobulin originated in the thyroid gland. This confirms that the autoimmune reaction that takes place in the thyroid is very similar to the autoimmune reaction that takes place in the eyes. It helps to bolster the argument in favor of using anti-immunity therapy for hyperthyroid eye disease, as I discuss in Chapter 6.

Goiters and Nodules

Goiters and nodules remain a very common problem in thyroid medicine. Newer studies are changing how doctors manage patients with these conditions.

Performing surgery after ethanol injections

One of the newer techniques for eliminating nodules in the thyroid is the injection of ethanol directly into the nodules (see Chapter 7). When this technique was brand-new, it raised the question of whether surgeons would face complications if they had to operate on patients who had ethanol injections. For example, a surgeon might need to operate if the ethanol failed to eliminate a nodule, if a doctor suspected that a nodule was malignant, or if a nodule were compressing a patient's trachea.

A study published in the periodical *Thyroid* in 2000 reported that surgeons did not encounter any special surgical problems while operating on the thyroids of 13 people who had previously been given ethanol injections.

The best assurance that ethanol injections don't cause problems down the road is to do your research and make certain that the person giving you an injection is highly skilled and experienced.

Shrinking goiters

Thyroid hormone has been used for decades to treat goiters; the hope has always been that the hormone will help to shrink the goiter. Most recent studies have shown that goiters respond little if at all to thyroid hormone.

In a study published in 2001 in the *Journal of Clinical Endocrinology and Metabolism* from the Netherlands, the authors compared thyroid hormone to radioactive iodine in the treatment of goiters. They used ultrasound to measure goiter size, and they measured the thyroid function of all test patients.

The researchers found that patients who received radioactive iodine had, on average, a 44 percent reduction in goiter size, while those who took thyroid hormone had a reduction of 1 percent. Only 1 of 29 patients didn't respond to radioactive iodine, while 16 of 28 had no response to thyroid hormone. Almost half the patients who got radioactive iodine developed hypothyroidism, while 10 of 28 taking thyroid hormone had symptoms of hyperthyroidism. In addition, those on thyroid hormone developed increased bone turnover and a loss of bone mineral density. The conclusion of this study is that radioactive iodine is more effective and better tolerated than thyroid hormone in the treatment of goiters.

If you have a goiter and want to get rid of it, you are much better off with radioactive iodine than thyroid hormone. The days of using thyroid hormone for this condition may be numbered.

New Approaches in Thyroid Cancer

Not surprisingly, much of the research concerning advances in thyroid disease centers around thyroid cancer. The following sections provide you with some of the more provocative and important studies of the last year or two. Undoubtedly, many more studies will come.

Understanding the impact of radioiodine exposure

More than 15 years after the nuclear disaster in Chernobyl, researchers still follow up with the children who were exposed to excessive radioactive iodine. In the *World Journal of Surgery* in 2000, a group of Russian scientists published the results of surgery on 330 children who had thyroid cancer after Chernobyl. The cancers tended to develop rapidly after exposure, were more aggressive than typical thyroid cancers, and had spread early to distant sites in the body. The patients were treated by *total thyroidectomy* (removal of the entire thyroid), followed by radioactive iodine treatment and suppression of TSH. The authors of the study emphasize that many more cases of thyroid cancer will be found among the children of Chernobyl, and they need to be monitored over the next several decades.

Are any environmental factors protective in the situation of radioactive iodine exposure? A study in *Environmental Health* in 2000 looked at people in Germany who were exposed to radioactive iodine. The study confirmed that drinking coffee and eating cruciferous vegetables like broccoli reduce the risk of developing cancer. If a patient had a goiter prior to the exposure, or if he consumed decaffeinated coffee instead of caffeinated, he was at increased risk for malignant or benign tumors.

These researchers also found that tomato consumption was a risk factor for malignant disease. They suggest that off-season tomatoes coming from areas where the farmers are careless about the use of chemicals may promote the development of thyroid cancer.

Blocking estrogen to slow tumor growth

One source of bewilderment about thyroid cancer is that it occurs more often in women than men. One study suggests that the reason may lie with the fact that women make estrogens as their primary sex hormone, and estrogen may stimulate thyroid tumor cell growth.

Writing in the 2001 *Journal of Clinical Endocrinology and Metabolism*, the authors of this study describe an experiment in which estrogen was shown to stimulate tumor cells and, to a lesser extent, benign cells. (Estrogen activates a metabolic pathway that leads to much greater growth activity in both malignant and benign cells.) When a drug that blocks estrogen action was given to patients, the tumor cells were no longer stimulated.

Predicting thyroid cancer

Is it possible to predict the future occurrence of thyroid cancer? In a study from Iceland, the authors present an analysis of blood that was taken many years before the diagnosis of thyroid cancer was made in 164 patients. Their study was published in *Acta Oncologica* in 2000.

The authors report that levels of *thyroglobulin*, the chemical that resides in the thyroid and is monitored when following thyroid cancer patients, could also be found in much elevated levels up to 15 years before the diagnosis of thyroid cancer was made. In contrast, there was no difference in the blood levels of TSH or thyroid hormone in the thyroid cancer patients compared to patients who never had thyroid cancer.

Detecting residual thyroid cancer

Another important recent advance is in the ability to detect thyroid cancer that remains after surgery. Thyroglobulin plays a major role in detecting remaining cancer. Another important tool that is often used is the whole body radioactive iodine scan, which can locate active thyroid tissue. The limitation of the scan is that it can't locate thyroid tissue that isn't making thyroid hormone. Sometimes a thyroglobulin level is high, indicating that active thyroid tissue is present, but the body scan is negative.

A newer type of scan called a *PET scan* is able to localize thyroid tissue that is not functioning well as thyroid tissue but is very metabolically active. A study in *Advances in Internal Medicine* in 2001 reviews the successful use of the PET scan for this purpose.

The study points out that the need still exists for new agents that attack these tumor tissues when they are discovered and that don't concentrate radioactive iodine.

If you have had thyroid cancer and discover a new growth that does not concentrate radioactive iodine on a thyroid scan, ask your doctor about the possibility of having a PET scan.

Following up thyroid cancer treatment

Does the thyroid cancer patient need to be followed for life, or is there a point at which the patient can be considered cured of the disease? The authors of a study in *Annales Chirurgiae* in 2000 attempt to answer this question.

The study's authors contend that it is necessary to study patients for seven months after they have had thyroid surgery. At that time, they can be divided into groups:

- ✓ **Group I:** Patients with microcancers

- ✓ **Group II:** Patients with no lymph node involvement or metastases, and normal thyroglobulin

    A: Younger than age 45

    B: Age 45 or older

- ✓ **Group III:** Patients with cancer with lymph node involvement but a normal thyroglobulin

- ✓ **Group IV:** Patients who have extension of the cancer beyond local lymph nodes or an elevated thyroglobulin

The survival rates for these groups are shown in Table 15-1.

Table 15-1	Survival Rates for Thyroid Cancer Patients	
Length of Time After Surgery	*10 Years*	*15 Years*
Group I	100 percent	100 percent
Group IIA	100 percent	100 percent

Length of Time After Surgery	10 Years	15 Years
Group IIB	96 percent	92 percent
Group III	100 percent	100 percent
Group IV	86 percent	73 percent

The latest time a recurrence was found in groups I and IIA was at 12 years. For groups IIB, III, and IV, tumors were discovered as late as 16 years after treatment. The study emphasizes that thyroglobulin tests and whole body scanning must be done every 5 years. Patients in groups I and IIA need to be followed for up to 15 years, while the other patients should be followed for 20 years before saying with certainty that the disease is eliminated. If a recurrence occurs, then the patient needs to be followed another 10 years with no more cancer before declaring that he or she is cancer-free.

Knowing what to expect from medullary thyroid cancer

Medullary thyroid cancer (MTC) is different from thyroid cell cancers like follicular or papillary cancer (see Chapter 8). MTC arises from the C-cells in the thyroid and can't be detected with radioactive iodine.

A study from Finland in the *Annales Chiarurgiae Gynecologica* in 2000 provides helpful information about the prognosis of medullary thyroid cancer. The authors divided their cases into hereditary (inherited) MTC and sporadic (not inherited) MTC. They found that sporadic MTC is a much deadlier disease than familial MTC.

Both groups were treated with total thyroidectomy and lymph node dissection. The group with sporadic MTC had a ten-year survival rate of 57.9 percent. Within the group of patients with sporadic MTC, those who had recurrent cancer in their lymph nodes, which was found and removed, had a survival rate of only 51.4 percent at ten years.

More important predictors of survival than lymph nodes were distant metastases and local spread of the cancer in the neck.

Using recombinant TSH with thyroid cancer patients

Recombinant TSH is a valuable tool both for the detection and treatment of residual thyroid cancer. Before recombinant TSH, in order to be tested for residual cancer with a total body scan, patients had to be taken off thyroid replacement hormone for four weeks or longer to allow their tissues to become hypothyroid. Going off hormone replacement greatly enhances the uptake of radioactive iodine, allowing for a more accurate scan of thyroid tissue.

Doctors have always been concerned that this time off the thyroid hormone allows cancer to grow more rapidly. For this reason, they use recombinant TSH to stimulate uptake and identify cancer recurrences without needing to stop taking thyroid hormone.

A group in Massachusetts, writing in the *Journal of Clinical Endocrinology and Metabolism* in 2001, explored the dosages of recombinant TSH required for optimal effect. They looked at patients' thyroglobulin levels, as well as TSH, T4, and T3. They found that a dose of 0.3 milligrams of recombinant TSH produced the maximal increase in thyroglobulin and radioactive iodine uptake. Going higher than 0.3 milligrams didn't increase the effect of treatment.

Another group from New York showed that using recombinant TSH was just as good as taking patients off thyroid medication in stimulating thyroglobulin secretion and radioactive iodine uptake. They concluded that preparing patients for a scan with recombinant TSH is equivalent to taking patients off thyroid hormone, in terms of diagnostic accuracy. Their work is found in the *European Journal of Endocrinology* in 2001.

Finally, recombinant TSH can be used to stimulate thyroid cancer to take up radioactive iodine in order to destroy it. In a study published in 2001 in the *European Journal of Endocrinology,* scientists used recombinant TSH to increase uptake. They noted that the recombinant TSH was free of side effects other than mild nausea. The results were excellent. The thyroid cancer treatment was as effective as with patients who were taken off thyroid hormone therapy prior to treatment. By using recombinant TSH, patients avoid the discomfort of being without thyroid hormone for weeks and avoid becoming hypothyroid.

Testing calcium levels after cancer surgery

In the process of removing the thyroid gland because of thyroid cancer, patients inevitably experience some trauma to the parathyroid glands that lie on the back of the thyroid lobes. Most of the time, these glands recover, but sometimes the trauma results in permanent hypoparathyroidism, which causes a patient to have low calcium levels.

In a study published in the *Journal of the European Society of Surgery and Oncology* in 2000, researchers wanted to establish how long it takes cancer patients to recover their normal calcium levels, as well as to determine how often treatment is necessary.

The study showed that if a patient had just one lobe of the thyroid removed, even though two of the parathyroid glands were not touched, there was a 10 percent drop in the level of calcium. Thirty-four percent of patients with this type of surgery required some calcium treatment because the level fell too low. Their calcium levels returned to normal within one week after surgery and remained normal.

When both sides of the thyroid were operated upon, as expected, there was more effect upon the parathyroids and the calcium. Calcium levels decreased 15 percent on average; some patients experienced severely low levels early in their recovery. The calcium decline was greater if the number of parathyroid glands that were preserved was fewer. Fifteen percent of these patients needed calcium treatment for two to seven days, 26 percent for eight to 180 days, and 9 percent for longer than a year. Only one patient of 82 required permanent treatment for low calcium after a single thyroid surgery on both sides, while one of four who had several thyroid surgeries needed permanent calcium treatment.

Tackling Iodine Deficiency Disease

When you consider the numbers of people affected by iodine deficiency disease (see Chapter 12), you would think that most of the papers in a search for articles on thyroid disease would concern themselves with this topic. However, the disease is not a common problem in the United States, so American scientists, who make up the majority of the world's investigators, don't tend to write about it. Still, plenty is going on in this area. This section describes the more important recent studies on iodine deficiency disease.

Recognizing the importance of selenium

Selenium is an element that plays a role in thyroid hormone production, because it is part of an enzyme responsible for converting T4 into T3. Until now, researchers and doctors have generally believed that selenium deficiency alone does not cause hypothyroidism; only when an iodine deficiency exists does selenium deficiency contribute to the disease. However, a study from the journal *Biological Trace Element Research* in 2000 contradicts this belief. The study's authors describe three girls who had hypothyroidism due to lack of selenium alone. When given replacement selenium, all returned to normal thyroid function. This study is the first description of hypothyroidism due to lack of selenium alone.

Using iodized oil for goiters

Iodized oil injection is commonly used to treat iodine deficiency and prevent goiter formation in areas of the world where iodine deficiency persists (see Chapter 12). The authors of a study in *Medicine* in 2001 wanted to consider any potential problems associated with lipiodol — a type of iodized oil. When lipiodol was given to a person who already had a multinodular goiter, that person sometimes became hyperthyroid. The hyperthyroidism tended to be mild and didn't last long. If the patient was a pregnant woman, the iodine sometimes entered the bloodstream of the fetus but was not found to cause a problem there.

The study confirms that using iodized oil for the replacement of iodine is a safe, cheap, and effective way to treat this deficiency.

Increasing the intelligence of babies born to hypothyroid mothers

Babies born to hypothyroid mothers tend to have low intelligence. In a study done in Taiwan and published in the *Journal of the Formosa Medical Association* in 2001, researchers looked at the level of intelligence of 62 babies of hypothyroid mothers and sought an early screening to avoid retardation. They found that the level of T4 at the time of diagnosis was a good predictor of the future intelligence of the baby. By measuring T4 at birth and giving replacement thyroid hormone, they could improve the outlook of these babies in terms of their intelligence.

As you can see, just about every aspect of thyroid disease is being studied, with articles in every medical journal. If you have a particular problem that concerns you or a loved one, don't hesitate to use the enormous, free resources at your disposal. Go to the Pub Med Web page mentioned at the beginning of this chapter (www.ncbi.nlm.nih.gov/PubMed), or check out your local bookstore and hospital library. And be sure to utilize the references you find in Appendix B of this book.

Chapter 16

The Thyroid and Pregnancy

In the last ten years, doctors have learned a lot about how the thyroid functions during pregnancy. This new level of understanding makes a tremendous difference in your ability to have a healthy baby, even if you have a thyroid disorder. If you and your doctor keep up with the latest information available, thyroid disease should not seriously impact your ability to have a healthy baby.

This chapter is about the wonderful state of pregnancy, with particular reference to how it changes thyroid function and how abnormalities of thyroid function affect the pregnancy. As I explain in earlier chapters, thyroid disease is very common among women. Many women come into a pregnancy with a thyroid condition, whether they know it or not. For the health of both the mother and the fetus, it's important to detect the condition and treat it appropriately. Some women develop a thyroid condition during pregnancy. This chapter explains how your thyroid function should be monitored during pregnancy and describes some of the consequences that could occur from not managing a thyroid condition.

The Normal Thyroid During Pregnancy

Three important changes occur in a woman's body during pregnancy, leading to a much greater need for iodine:

✔ Early in pregnancy, the flow of blood to her kidneys is increased, resulting in more clearing of iodine and a greater loss of iodine through the urine.

✔ Because the fetus cannot make thyroid hormone at first, it takes thyroid hormone from the mother through the placenta.

✔ The growing fetus starts to make its own thyroid hormone after a while and needs iodine to do so.

At the same time, as a result of increases in hormones, particularly estrogen, the mother makes much more thyroxine-binding globulin — a protein that transports thyroid hormone through the blood — than she used to. She also makes a form of thyroxine-binding globulin that leaves the circulation much more slowly. This substance takes up a lot of the thyroid hormone that the mother's body is making, which leads to an even greater need for iodine to make more.

If you are hypothyroid and take thyroid hormone pills, it's important to understand all these changes. To maintain normal thyroid function, your dose of thyroid hormone replacement will probably need to be increased early in pregnancy, based upon your level of thyroid-stimulating hormone (TSH).

While all these changes are happening, the placenta — the tissue that connects the fetus to the mother — is making a lot of a hormone called *human chorionic gonadotrophin* (HCG). HCG has some parts that look very much like TSH. It reaches the mother's thyroid and starts to stimulate it into making more thyroid hormone, just as TSH would do. As a result, the mother's level of free T4 rises, causing a fall in the amount of TSH her body produces. If she is having twins, her HCG level can be especially high and can persist for weeks. As I show you later in this chapter, the result may be a form of hyperthyroidism.

One of the confusing aspects of pregnancy, with respect to thyroid disease, is that many signs and symptoms of a normal pregnancy are similar to the findings in hyperthyroidism. These signs and symptoms include:

✔ A rapid heart rate

✔ Intolerance to heat

✔ Tiredness

✔ Anxiety

✔ Trouble sleeping

✔ Sweating

Your weight is the biggest clue as to whether hyperthyroidism is an issue. Most pregnant women gain weight throughout their pregnancy (although some women lose a few pounds initially if they experience vomiting). A hyperthyroid woman often does not gain weight, and sometimes loses weight, during pregnancy.

Pregnancy and Hypothyroidism

It is a miracle that a mother's body does not reject a fetus as a foreign intruder, just as it would reject any foreign invasion. (Even a few foreign cells injected inside your body wouldn't last long.)

The fact that the mother's body doesn't reject the fetus is evidence that a general decline in immunity takes place during pregnancy. As a result, women who have autoimmune diseases prior to pregnancy often discover that they improve during a pregnancy, with the condition returning to its original state again after delivery. This is true for people with either hypothyroidism or hyperthyroidism that results from an autoimmune condition.

Decreased fertility

If a woman has hypothyroidism that is not treated, she will probably have a difficult time becoming pregnant because the hypothyroidism decreases her fertility. (In a study of infertile women in Finland, published in *Gynecological Endocrinology* in 2000, five percent were found to be hypothyroid.)

If the hypothyroid woman does become pregnant, the risk of a miscarriage is much higher than if she didn't have a thyroid condition.

If you suffer one or more miscarriages, be sure to have your doctor check your thyroid function.

If you are hypothyroid and are not being treated with thyroid hormone replacement, you may suffer from a number of obstetric complications if you become pregnant. Complications may include high blood pressure, problems with the placental connection to the fetus, and problems with delivery. All this is avoided with proper treatment of the thyroid.

Iodine deficiency

A mother with an iodine deficiency during pregnancy cannot make sufficient thyroid hormone for herself and her fetus. (The fetus gets the thyroid hormone it needs from its mother up until the 20th week of the pregnancy.) As a result, the mother will be chronically stimulated by TSH to make more thyroid hormone, and she will develop a goiter.

A goiter does not develop in the mother during a normal pregnancy. If a mother develops a goiter, it means that she is experiencing iodine deficiency, hypothyroidism, or hyperthyroidism.

The mother's goiter may not fully shrink after delivery, when her iodine needs are reduced. This may partly explain the much greater incidence of thyroid enlargement in women when compared with men.

The fetus is also strongly affected by iodine deficiency. It may develop a goiter as well, and it may suffer from abnormal brain development (see Chapter 12). A goiter in the fetus could result in problems during delivery.

Laboratory tests show that iodine-deficient pregnant women have:

- ✔ Reduced T4 and, if severe, reduced T3 hormone levels
- ✔ Increased TSH
- ✔ Increased ratios of T3 to T4, because the thyroid begins to prefer making T3
- ✔ Increased thyroglobulin

Autoimmune hypothyroidism

Autoimmune thyroid disease is much more common in iodine-rich countries than in iodine-deficient countries. Most cases of hypothyroidism in pregnancy result from this disease.

Understanding the risks to the mother and fetus

If lab tests show that a woman has thyroid autoantibodies — even if she is not diagnosed as hypothyroid because her thyroid function tests are normal — she is at an increased risk for a miscarriage. Doctors are not clear why this is so. One suggestion is that these women really have mild hypothyroidism despite the normal test results. Another is that the autoantibodies are just a marker for other autoimmune diseases that may be responsible for the miscarriage. A third hypothesis is that miscarriage in these autoimmune mothers is meant to prevent the transmission of autoimmune diseases to the next generation.

The thyroid autoantibodies can be transmitted to the fetus through the placenta, causing hypothyroidism in the fetus. Usually, if the mother is hypothyroid and is being adequately treated with thyroid hormone, enough gets to the fetus to prevent this problem. If the baby is born with hypothyroidism, he or she can be placed on thyroid hormone replacement until the autoantibodies are cleared from the baby's circulation, usually in three or four months. The baby does not need treatment after that.

Knowing when to treat the mother

At what point is treatment needed for autoimmune hypothyroidism in pregnancy? If a mother's TSH level is greater than 4, it is appropriate to treat her. She needs to have thyroid function tests during every trimester of pregnancy to confirm that she is receiving the right amount of thyroid medication.

If the mother's TSH level is between 2 and 4, and she tests positive for thyroid autoantibodies, she should probably be treated and the fetus should be checked for goiter or other signs of a thyroid abnormality. Fortunately, recent studies show that if the mother has very mild hypothyroidism in early pregnancy, it has no negative effect upon the newborn's hearing or physical activity.

Although autoimmune hypothyroidism generally improves during pregnancy, after the baby is born, the mother's hypothyroidism may become worse and her T4 level may decrease further. Her TSH should be checked every six to eight weeks after delivery.

If you have hypothyroidism during pregnancy, be sure to have thyroid function tests done about two months after delivery to verify that you are taking the right dose of thyroid hormone.

Certain drugs that are commonly taken during pregnancy, such as iron, sucralfate, and aluminum hydroxide (see Chapter 10), can block the absorption of thyroid hormone. These drugs should be taken several hours before or after the thyroid hormone is taken.

Hyperthyroidism in Pregnancy

Doctors once believed that most hyperthyroidism in pregnancy was due to Graves' disease. Recently, it has become clear that there is another cause for hyperthyroidism in pregnancy that is actually more frequent than Graves' disease — a condition called *gestational transient thyrotoxicosis.* I discuss both conditions in this section.

Regardless of the cause, the symptoms of hyperthyroidism in pregnancy are those mentioned earlier in this chapter: rapid heart rate, sweating, trouble sleeping, anxiety, heat intolerance, and fatigue. These symptoms are all fairly common for any pregnant woman. One way to determine whether the mother is hyperthyroid is that if she has Graves' disease, she will usually not gain a great deal of weight during pregnancy; she may even lose weight.

Lab tests show that a hyperthyroid mother has high levels of free T4 and low levels of TSH. In this situation, doing a total T4 test (see Chapter 4) is not helpful at all, because the total T4 will always be elevated in view of the increase in thyroid-binding globulin in the mother's system.

Hyperthyroidism needs to be controlled during pregnancy. If it is not controlled, some of the consequences may include:

- Premature delivery
- Fetal malformations
- Low birth weight
- Hyperthyroidism in the infant
- High blood pressure and other problems in the mother

Graves' disease

Alice Dummy is a cousin of Stacy, Karen, Sarah, and Margaret — our friends from earlier chapters. She is married, but — conveniently for us — she kept her maiden name. She became pregnant about a month ago. She notices that her heart is beating very fast all the time and that she is feeling very warm. She has actually lost a few pounds. Her husband notices that her neck seems enlarged.

Alice and her husband go to their obstetrician, Dr. Ufbaum, who obtains thyroid blood tests to rule out hyperthyroidism. To her surprise, Dr. Ufbaum rules *in* the possibility of hyperthyroidism when she finds that the free T4 level in Alice's blood is elevated while the TSH level is suppressed. The doctor immediately refers Alice to her favorite endocrinologist, Dr. Rubin.

Dr. Rubin sends Alice for a blood test for thyroid-stimulating hormone receptor stimulating antibodies. The test result is very positive. He starts Alice on the antithyroid medication propylthiouricil. Within three weeks, Alice begins to feel better. By six weeks, she is gaining weight and her heart has slowed noticeably. It is actually possible to take Alice off the propylthiouricil during the second half of her pregnancy, which proceeds normally. Dr. Rubin instructs Dr. Ufbaum to check carefully for hyperthyroidism in the fetus; fortunately, it does not develop.

After the delivery, Alice again needs antithyroid medication, which she takes for a year. She does well.

The development of hyperthyroidism during a pregnancy is relatively uncommon. It is believed to occur in no more than 2 of every 1,000 pregnancies.

This type of hyperthyroidism is associated with antibodies that stimulate the TSH receptors on thyroid cells and trigger the production of more thyroid hormone. In some cases, the mother may have had Graves' disease prior to pregnancy and been successfully treated with radioactive iodine, surgery, or antithyroid drugs. She may have normal thyroid function, but she still has the antibodies that can be transferred through the placenta to the fetus, giving the fetus hyperthyroidism and a probable goiter.

Finding hyperthyroidism in the fetus

A number of signs indicate that the fetus has hyperthyroidism, most of which are determined by an ultrasound study of the developing fetus. They include:

- ✔ Fetal goiter
- ✔ Very rapid fetal heart rate (over 160 beats per minute)
- ✔ Increased movement of the fetus
- ✔ Acceleration in the bone maturity of the fetus
- ✔ Fetal growth retardation

If you become pregnant after successful treatment for Graves' disease, your fetus can become hyperthyroid because you still have thyroid-stimulating antibodies that can pass through the placenta. It is important for your doctor to monitor the fetus for signs of hyperthyroidism and check you for TSH receptor antibodies early in pregnancy. If your TSH receptor antibodies are elevated, but there are no signs of fetal hyperthyroidism, both should be checked again in six months.

Treatment of hyperthyroidism in the fetus is accomplished by giving antithyroid drugs to the mother; the medication passes through the placenta to decrease the thyroid function of the fetus. The mother may need to also take thyroid hormone replacement, because her thyroid function will be reduced by the antithyroid drugs as well.

The fetus may also show hyperthyroidism at birth if the mother has Graves' disease that has not been well controlled or has a lot of TSH receptor stimulating antibodies. A mother who has previously had a baby with neonatal hyperthyroidism is at especially high risk to have another in a subsequent pregnancy.

Hyperthyroidism in the newborn may not appear until the antithyroid drugs, obtained through the placenta, have cleared out of the baby's system. The baby will then have the usual signs of hyperthyroidism plus signs specific to a newborn, such as failure to thrive, increase in the yellow color of the skin (due to increased bilirubin), and increased irritability. After the mother's thyroid-stimulating antibodies are cleared from the baby's blood, the baby will have normal thyroid function.

Treating the mother during pregnancy

As I mention earlier in the chapter, autoimmune hyperthyroidism tends to improve through the course of a pregnancy because there is a general decline in the mother's autoimmunity. Other factors aiding the improvement of autoimmune hyperthyroidism include an increase in thyroxine-binding globulin, an increased loss of iodine in the urine, and an increase in TSH receptor blocking antibodies as the TSH receptor stimulating antibodies decline.

Radioactive iodine is not used to treat Graves' disease during a pregnancy, because the radiation could create malformations in the fetus and destroy the fetal thyroid gland.

The usual treatment for Graves' disease during pregnancy is the use of antithyroid drugs. At one time, propylthiouricil was preferred because it was thought that it did not cross the placenta, while methimazole did. However, methimazole is used in Europe and Asia without any problem, so most specialists feel that either one can be used.

The dose of antithyroid drug that is used is the least amount that can keep the free T4 in the upper part of the normal range (see Chapter 4). When this is done, the fetus receives the right amount of T4 from the mother.

A study of goiters in babies at birth found that 8 of 11 were due to hypothyroidism in the baby, while 3 were due to hyperthyroidism. Of the 8 hypothyroid babies, 5 were a result of excessive amounts of antithyroid drugs that were given to the mother during pregnancy. This emphasizes how important it is to give the least amount of antithyroid drug that can make the mother normal.

A few circumstances require surgery rather than antithyroid drugs, including the following:

- The patient fails to take the antithyroid drug.
- The mother needs exceptionally high doses of medication — more than 300 milligrams of propylthiouricil or 20 milligrams of methimazole daily.
- A slow fetal heart rate indicates that the fetus may be hypothyroid due to the antithyroid drug the mother is taking.

   ✔ The mother has extremely severe hyperthyroid symptoms.

   ✔ The mother experiences side effects, like a fall in white blood cells, from the drug.

If surgery must be performed, it is best done in the second trimester of the pregnancy, when it is least harmful to the fetus and the mother.

To prepare for surgery, the mother is sometimes given iodine. Iodine passes easily through the placenta to the fetus, where it can cause goiter and hypothyroidism. Iodine is also found in topical compounds and dyes used for better observation of the growing fetus. The use of iodine is necessary in these situations, but you should be aware of (and talk with your doctor about) the consequences of their use.

Checking mother and child after birth

The easiest way to check the thyroid status of a newborn is to check the levels of free T4 and TSH in the umbilical cord serum. Treatment will depend upon the findings.

After you deliver your baby, if your Graves' disease was under control during the pregnancy, you can expect a worsening of symptoms as the autoimmunity becomes severe again. It is important to check your thyroid function with blood tests after the delivery.

Postpartum Graves' disease is not the same as postpartum thyroiditis (see Chapter 11). The treatment for these two conditions is entirely different. Postpartum thyroiditis is a condition associated with a low uptake of radioactive iodine and results when a damaged thyroid spills thyroid hormone (rather than from stimulation by TSH receptor stimulating antibodies). Thyroglobulin also spills into the blood in postpartum thyroiditis but not in postpartum Graves' disease.

Postpartum thyroiditis is associated with a finding of thyroid autoantibodies. Some specialists recommend that all pregnant women have tests for thyroid autoantibodies early in pregnancy, because about 50 percent of those with positive tests will develop postpartum thyroiditis.

Breastfeeding with Graves' disease

For many years, doctors believed that mothers who were being treated with antithyroid drugs for Graves' disease should not breastfeed because the drugs would enter her milk and pass to the baby. Recent studies have proved that this is not the case.

One study showed that there was no effect on breastfed infants when the mothers were taking up to 750 milligrams of propylthiouricil (PTU) daily. In another study, the same thing was found when the mothers were taking up to 20 milligrams of methimazole daily.

You can breastfeed safely if you are taking antithyroid drugs for hyperthyroidism. Use the guidelines in the previous paragraph for the maximum dosage of drugs.

Gestational transient thyrotoxicosis

Holly Bright is a 27-year-old woman who has become pregnant for the first time. She has had a lot of morning sickness during the first several weeks of her pregnancy. She notices that she has lost some weight, but she believes that it is due to the morning sickness. However, in the last few days, she has had symptoms of a rapid heartbeat, fatigue, trouble sleeping, and a feeling of warmth all the time. She checks with her obstetrician, Dr. Ufbaum. As a result of her recent experience with Alice Dummy, Dr. Ufbaum is convinced that Holly has Graves' disease. Thyroid function tests seem to confirm this. She refers Holly to Dr. Rubin.

Dr. Rubin is not as convinced. He notices that her thyroid is not enlarged. He is concerned about the extent of the vomiting that Holly describes. He sends her to be tested for TSH receptor stimulating autoantibodies. The result is negative. Dr. Rubin tells Holly that she probably has a condition called *gestational transient thyrotoxicosis.* He is able to reassure her that the condition will be brief. He gives her a low dose of propranolol, a drug that relieves her symptoms, along with a drug for her vomiting. Over the next few weeks, Holly returns to normal and has no further trouble with hyperthyroid symptoms. The thyroid function tests also return to normal.

Gestational transient thyrotoxicosis (GTT) is actually more common than Graves' disease in pregnancy, occurring as often as two to three times in 100 pregnancies. Fortunately, it is generally mild. But it's sometimes more serious, and it can be confused with Graves' disease, leading to incorrect treatment.

GTT is caused by the hormone called *human chorionic gonadotrophin* (HCG), which I discuss in the section "The Normal Thyroid During Pregnancy" earlier in the chapter. HCG is at its highest level in the mother's circulation at around ten weeks of pregnancy, but it continues to be elevated above normal throughout. It may appear in a form that is cleared very slowly from the circulation of the mother. It can act as a stimulant on the thyroid, leading to increased free T4 and decreased TSH, which produces a diagnosis of hyperthyroidism. No TSH receptor stimulating antibodies are found in GTT.

About half of GTT patients show the typical symptoms of hyperthyroidism. In addition, many patients experience a significant increase in vomiting associated with this condition, sometimes called *hyperemesis gravidarum*. A goiter is not usually found in patients with GTT.

Most patients need no more treatment than beta blockers like propranolol (see Chapter 6). Sometimes the mother has to be given fluids to replenish what she loses from vomiting. Occasionally, antithyroid drugs need to be given for a short time, until levels of HCG begin to fall (usually after ten weeks of pregnancy). However, in twin pregnancies, HCG levels may be particularly high and sustained for a longer time period. Some studies have not shown a difference in the level of HCG between pregnant women who vomit a lot and those who do not. This suggests that women who experience a lot of vomiting may be making a form of HCG that is especially stimulating to the thyroid.

The most severe vomiting associated with GTT occurs when the level of thyroid hormone, the level of HCG, and the level of estrogen in the pregnant mother are all at a maximum.

If you have symptoms of hyperthyroidism accompanied by vomiting early in pregnancy, your doctor should consider GTT as the diagnosis rather than Graves' disease. GTT can be expected to pass after several weeks, while Graves' disease will require treatment throughout the pregnancy in many cases.

Hydatidiform mole and choriocarcinoma

Occasionally, as a result of some abnormality of the mother's egg or in fertilization, the placenta forms a series of grape-like clusters called a *hydatidiform mole*. No viable fetus can result from this mole, but in about 10 percent of cases it can secrete large amounts of HCG and cause hyperthyroidism. The mother often experiences vaginal bleeding, and her uterus is not the correct size for the stage of the pregnancy (it is usually too large).

An ultrasound study is often performed in this situation, showing the mole very clearly. Because there is no viable fetus, the pregnancy is terminated.

Very rarely — about 2 percent of the time — the mole changes into a cancer called a *choriocarcinoma,* which also can make a large amount of HCG. Fortunately, this cancer is very treatable, and the patient may even be able to preserve the ability to have children.

New Thyroid Nodules in Pregnancy

Because pregnant women have frequent exams and are followed carefully, thyroid nodules are sometimes discovered during pregnancy. Treatment depends upon the tissue found in the nodule and the stage of the pregnancy.

The first step is to do a fine needle aspiration biopsy of the nodule (see Chapter 7). If the biopsy shows that a nodule is definitely cancer, and the patient hasn't yet reached her third trimester, she should have surgery of the thyroid at that time. The second trimester is the best time for this surgery because it offers the least chance of interfering with the development of the baby or causing premature labor.

If the biopsy does not definitely show cancer, it is safe to wait until after the delivery, when a radioactive iodine scan is done (see Chapter 4). Keep in mind that after a radioactive scan is done, the mother cannot breastfeed her baby. If the scan shows that the iodine uptake is high, the nodule probably isn't cancer. If the scan shows that the nodule remains cold, and the diagnosis remains uncertain, then surgery is done to obtain a final diagnosis and determine the appropriate treatment.

Some evidence exists that pregnancy and breastfeeding tend to stimulate the development of a new thyroid cancer if the woman is less than 45 years of age. There is no association between the number of births, the age during the first birth, or the age during the last birth and the incidence of thyroid cancer if the woman is over 45, according to one study.

Chapter 17

Thyroid Conditions and Children

● ●

In This Chapter

▶ Understanding thyroid function in newborns and infants

▶ Screening for thyroid disease in babies

▶ Dealing with hypo- and hyperthyroidism in kids

▶ Concentrating on goiters

▶ Treating thyroid nodules in the young

● ●

*N*ewborns and children who have thyroid abnormalities present special problems because their brains and bodies are developing at the same time that their thyroids aren't functioning properly. Thyroid hormones are a critical part of their development. The hormones must be available in the right amount at the right time in order for a child to have normal mental function and normal growth.

Children can experience all the kinds of thyroid diseases that are seen in adults. This chapter discusses normal thyroid development and the impact of thyroid diseases on a developing human being. As a parent, you can do little to treat these conditions, but your early recognition of a problem, your understanding of the consequences if the problem is not treated, and your continued support of your child through treatment and recovery can have a major impact on the way your child handles this challenge.

Understanding the Onset of Thyroid Function

First, a quick review. Thyroid hormones (T3 and T4) are produced when *thyroid-stimulating hormone* (TSH) stimulates the thyroid to make them. TSH is released from the pituitary gland when the hypothalamus produces *thyrotrophin-releasing hormone* (TRH). All these structures and their hormones are in place when a baby is born. Much recent research has established how this process comes about.

After just 15 weeks of development, the fetus shows function in its pituitary gland, and TRH can be detected. TSH and the other pituitary hormones start to appear between weeks 10 and 17. The thyroid is functioning by the 10th week, and its production of thyroid hormone becomes significant around the 20th week. The ability of thyroid hormone to shut off TSH production matures towards the end of the pregnancy and in the first two months after delivery.

The placenta acts as a barrier, preventing the mother's TSH from reaching the circulation of the fetus throughout the pregnancy. The placenta also contains an enzyme that breaks down the mother's thyroid hormones before they can reach the fetus. In breaking down the hormones, the enzyme releases iodine from the mother's hormones so the fetus can use the iodine to make thyroid hormone for itself. At the same time, the placenta is producing *human chorionic gonadotrophin,* a hormone that stimulates the thyroid (see Chapter 16).

As the pregnancy progresses, the enzyme in the placenta that breaks down the mother's thyroid hormones stops working as much, and other enzymes take over to convert T4 into the active hormone, T3. By not working so much, the placental enzyme no longer prevents the mother's T4 from getting to the fetus. This is very important, because the fetus needs the T4 for normal development, especially of its brain, at a time when it cannot make much T4 for itself.

One enzyme, which converts T4 to T3, works in the liver, the kidneys, and the thyroid. Another enzyme works mainly in the pituitary gland. If the fetus is not getting enough T4, the enzyme in the pituitary increases, and the other one decreases so the fetal brain gets enough T3.

While the baby is born, leaving the warmth of the uterus for the colder temperatures of the outside world, the baby's pituitary releases a large amount of TSH. This stimulates the thyroid to release a large amount of T3 and T4, causing the temperature of the baby's body to rise. This process is known as the *TSH surge*. The TSH surge peaks after only 30 minutes but continues to stimulate extra thyroid hormone for the next 24 hours.

A premature baby has similar hormone changes to a normal-term baby, but to a lesser extent. It does not have as much of a TSH surge and does not produce as much thyroid hormone. The T3 does not increase as much either, because the converting enzymes are not yet as active. This baby cannot defend its body temperature the way that a normal-term baby can.

As the baby grows, it stores more thyroid hormones in its thyroid along with thyroglobulin (see Chapter 3), and it produces more thyroid hormone. The thyroid gland grows so the lobes are normally about the same size as the part of the baby's thumbs after the last joint (the *terminal phalanx*).

A lack of thyroid hormone during fetal growth has important consequences (see Chapter 12). Thyroid hormone is particularly important in the development of hearing, but many other body organs also need it for proper development. Some of the damage that results from lack of thyroid hormone includes the following:

- ✔ Immature bones
- ✔ Immature liver
- ✔ Reduced mental function
- ✔ Increased sleepiness

The brain is dependent on thyroid hormone for development for the first two to three years after birth. For every month that thyroid hormone is not given to a hypothyroid newborn, he or she suffers a loss of five IQ points.

During the first 20 years of life, the free T3 and free T4 slowly decline, as does the total T3 and total T4 (see Chapter 3 for an explanation of the difference between *free* and *total*). As estrogen levels begin to rise during puberty in the female, her body makes more thyroid-binding globulin, and there's more total T3 and total T4. The decrease in the free T3 and free T4 is probably because of a gradual decline in TSH.

Screening the Newborn

Noah Stern is the newborn son of Barry and Sally Stern. Sally finds that Noah feeds very poorly. He seems to be cold to the touch. Otherwise he appears fine.

According to law, Noah is screened for hypothyroidism a couple days after birth. The TSH level comes back elevated at 35. The pediatrician notifies the Sterns and asks them to bring Noah in for testing. A blood test confirms that his TSH is elevated, and the free T4 is low. The pediatrician diagnoses congenital hypothyroidism.

A thyroid scan is performed on Noah, which shows little active thyroid tissue. Noah is given thyroid hormone, and his feeding and his body temperature rapidly improve. Sally notices that Noah looks less puffy as well. The doctor measures thyroid functions frequently until Noah stabilizes. Noah grows and feeds normally. He does not appear to have any deficits in his intellectual development.

The major reason for screening for thyroid disease is to diagnose congenital hypothyroidism as early as possible. *Congenital hypothyroidism* means hypothyroidism that is present when the baby is born (see the next section).

Because the consequences of not treating hypothyroidism in newborns are so great and the response to early treatment is so successful, screening for thyroid disease is considered to be essential in the newborn. In a study of 800 children who had congenital hypothyroidism before the era of screening began in 1974, the average IQ was 80, which is low. Some of these babies were noted to have signs of hypothyroidism and were tested. Children who were found by testing to have hypothyroidism and were treated appropriately experienced no lowering of the IQ. Within that group, some children were not adequately treated. Even these children had normal IQs, though somewhat lower than the fully treated children.

Screening is a simple process. A drop of blood is placed on filter paper. (This filter paper is the same type that is used for screening tests for other diseases as well.) Then the filter paper is tested for TSH (sometimes for T4 instead). If the TSH is above 40, the baby has a regular blood test for TSH and free T4, and the doctor begins treating the baby with thyroid hormone while waiting for the result. If the TSH is between 20 and 39, blood tests are done, but no treatment is begun until the diagnosis is confirmed. The reason is that up to 75 percent of babies with a TSH at this level during screening will test normal when a regular blood test is done.

A TSH surge occurs immediately after birth. Screening on the first day may result in a false positive test.

The screening test is not perfect. Children who have *secondary hypothyroidism,* which results from the body's failure to secrete TSH, will be missed. Screening also won't identify children who have a normal TSH and a low T4 (which is not being measured in the screening) at birth, whose TSH becomes abnormal a week later. Premature babies, especially, may show this pattern. Babies who fail to secrete TSH often have failure of other hormones as well, which leads to many signs and symptoms that point to disease.

Infants with low birth weight can be misdiagnosed because they tend to be born with low levels of hormones that soon rise to normal.

Screening has shown that congenital hypothyroidism is more common than was previously thought; about 1 in 3,750 babies are affected. Screening is now done, by law, throughout the United States and in Western Europe, Japan, Australia, New Zealand, and Israel. A major campaign is underway to promote neonatal screening for thyroid disease throughout the world.

Not only does screening make excellent medical sense, it makes excellent economic sense as well. A study in Denmark found that the future medical costs for the babies who were found to be positive at screening, had they not been discovered and treated, would have been 28 times the cost of screening all the babies in Denmark.

Coping with Hypothyroidism in Children

A number of conditions can cause hypothyroidism in the newborn and in the older child. You find out about these conditions in this section.

Specialists disagree as to whether pregnant mothers should be routinely tested for hypothyroidism to protect their babies from a hypothyroid environment. A study in the *New England Journal of Medicine* showed that babies experienced some slight loss of IQ if their mothers were hypothyroid and untreated during pregnancy. My own bias is that every pregnant woman should be screened for hypothyroidism with a TSH test.

Transient congenital hypothyroidism

Some babies are diagnosed with hypothyroidism at birth because their TSH levels are found to be high, but these levels fall to normal shortly after birth. This condition is called *transient congenital hypothyroidism* because it doesn't last. One common cause of this condition is iodine deficiency in the mother.

This condition is especially prevalent in very low-birth-weight infants, who should be screened for thyroid disease not only at birth, but also at 2 weeks and 6 weeks of age.

Because this condition is so common in premature infants, the question is whether these babies need thyroid supplementation for a short time at birth. A study in the *Texas Medical Journal* in 2000 suggests that babies who have more than 27 weeks gestation at the time of birth don't need supplemental thyroid hormone at birth and may actually be harmed by such treatment, whereas babies who spend less than 27 weeks in the uterus may benefit from supplementation.

Sometimes, determining whether the hypothyroidism is transient or permanent isn't possible. In this case, the baby is treated with thyroid hormone until the age of 4, and then treatment is stopped for a short time to see if the child can make his or her own thyroid hormone. This does not damage the child's brain.

Congenital hypothyroidism

Babies who are born with hypothyroidism that doesn't correct itself shortly after birth have *congenital hypothyroidism*. This condition used to be a significant cause of mental retardation, but when neonatal thyroid screening was begun in the 1970s, doctors were able to prevent mental retardation from occurring.

Causes

There are many causes of congenital hypothyroidism, but 80 percent of cases result from *thyroid dysgenesis* — a failure of the thyroid to grow or to end up in its proper place in the neck. Thyroid dysgenesis may be caused by:

- ✔ No thyroid at all (a condition called *thyroid agenesis*)
- ✔ A small gland that can't make enough thyroid hormone *(thyroid hypoplasia)*
- ✔ A thyroid gland that grows in the wrong place, often at the base of the tongue *(ectopic thyroid)*

Some of the other, far less frequent causes of congenital hypothyroidism include the following:

- ✔ The baby's thyroid doesn't respond to TSH.
- ✔ The mother is exposed to radioactive iodine that destroys the baby's thyroid.
- ✔ The hypothalamus does not release TRH (a condition called *hypothalamic hypothyroidism*).
- ✔ Some step of the synthesis of thyroid hormone is defective.

With the exception of maternal exposure to radioactive iodine, these conditions are all genetic diseases (see Chapter 14). In the United States, these diseases are rare among African-Americans and more frequent among Hispanics.

Signs and symptoms

Many babies with congenital hypothyroidism have few signs or symptoms of hypothyroidism at birth. This condition is discovered by screening (see "Screening the Newborn," earlier in the chapter). If the condition is severe, the baby shows some or all of the following signs:

- ✔ Low body temperature
- ✔ Slow heart rate
- ✔ Poor feeding
- ✔ Umbilical hernia (an outward protrusion of the umbilicus — the belly button — that may contain intestine)

Once the condition is recognized and confirmed, treatment should begin immediately. Doing a thyroid scan just before treating the baby may help detect any functioning thyroid tissue, a lack of which indicates the need for lifelong treatment. Tissue may not be seen, or tissue may be found in an unusual site. If no tissue is seen on the thyroid scan, a thyroid ultrasound will show whether tissue exists and whether it's unable to take up iodine possibly due to a genetic abnormality. This information can be helpful in counseling the parents about hypothyroidism in future children.

Treatment

Babies with congenital hypothyroidism are usually given a relatively high dose of thyroxine (T4) hormone replacement for the first week to restore their thyroid hormone levels. The daily dose administered after that initial dose must be individualized.

The baby's thyroid function should be checked at 7, 14, and 28 days. In view of all the changes taking place in thyroid function soon after birth, the stabilization of thyroid function may take time. Once the tests are normal and stable, they are measured every 3 months until 2 years of age and then every year.

Proper dosing of thyroid hormone is determined not only by taking thyroid-function tests but also by making sure that the baby is growing properly. The height and weight of the baby are checked regularly to verify the hormone dosage.

If thyroid hormone treatment is delayed more than 4 to 8 weeks after birth, a child with congenital hypothyroidism will almost certainly have some decrease in intellectual function.

Acquired hypothyroidism

Children may acquire hypothyroidism at any time after birth. When hypothyroidism occurs in a child over the age of 2, it does not damage brain function, but it does greatly affect growth and development.

Causes

Children may develop hypothyroidism for all the same reasons that adults become hypothyroid. Iodine deficiency is, by far, the most common cause throughout the world. Where iodine is sufficient, autoimmune thyroiditis (see Chapter 5) is the leading cause. Less common reasons for acquired hypothyroidism include:

✔ Drugs like iodine or lithium

✔ Irradiation — externally (for a tumor, for example) or internally, in treatment of hyperthyroidism with radioactive iodine

✔ Removal of the thyroid for any reason

✔ Abnormal production of thyroid hormone

✔ Resistance to thyroid hormone

✔ Central or secondary hypothyroidism due to a tumor in the pituitary or hypothalamus or a lack of production of TSH or TRH

Signs and symptoms

Again, the findings in these conditions are similar to the signs and symptoms found in adults, except that a growing, developing child experiences the consequences of poor growth. Constipation and dry skin are a feature of any hypothyroid person. The child, in addition, does not keep up with height and weight guidelines for growing children.

The child who becomes hypothyroid after he or she has entered school will start to have trouble with schoolwork or keeping up with the physical activity of the other children. Lack of energy is a major complaint at this time.

Interestingly, some of these kids appear unusually muscular, despite being weak. This is because they have swelling of their muscle fibers, which is called *pseudohypertrophy* of muscles.

The growth of the skeleton and the teeth is delayed. Other signs include:

✔ Enlarged thyroid (goiter), unless it has been removed

✔ Dry, cool skin that is puffy, pale, and yellowish

✔ Brittle nails and dry, brittle hair that tends to fall out excessively

✔ Swelling that does not retain an indentation, especially of the legs

✔ Hoarseness and slow speech with a thickened tongue

✔ An expressionless face

✔ A slow pulse

Some of these children occasionally show early sexual development. This is thought to be the result of the large amount of TSH in their bodies. TSH has a structure that shares some features with *follicle-stimulating hormone* (FSH). The TSH activates cells that would normally respond to FSH, so girls may have early vaginal bleeding, and boys may have large testicles for their age. The boys do not have a lot of male hormone, which is the result of stimulation by another hormone, *luteinizing hormone* (LH). TSH does not share features with LH. The girls, however, do have increased estrogen for their age since their ovaries can respond to the FSH-like properties of TSH; LH-like stimulation is not needed to accomplish this.

The adolescent who develops hypothyroidism has signs and symptoms that parallel the symptoms found in an adult, with a few differences. If the child has begun puberty, it may stop unless the child is given thyroid hormone treatment. Also, the growth of permanent teeth may be delayed, and the child doesn't gain height as quickly as would be expected.

When central or secondary hypothyroidism (a lack of TRH or TSH) is the cause, the signs and symptoms of hypothyroidism tend to be milder. The main symptoms are due to the underlying cause, which may be a brain tumor, for example. The child complains of headaches or trouble with vision.

Laboratory confirmation

A TSH and free T4 test will confirm the diagnosis of hypothyroidism. In order to make a diagnosis of chronic (autoimmune) thyroiditis, the child is tested for the presence of thyroid autoantibodies. The child's bone age is determined by X-rays to evaluate any growth abnormalities.

If central hypothyroidism is responsible, the free T4 and the TSH will be low, as will the other hormones made by the pituitary gland. An X-ray of the pituitary will be necessary to look for a tumor.

Treatment

The current treatment for hypothyroidism is thyroxine (T4) hormone replacement. However, recent studies suggest that giving both T3 and T4 replacement, in the same proportions that are made by the normal thyroid, may be more appropriate (see Chapter 5). This conclusion is based on studies in adults. Similar studies in children have not been published.

In most cases, the dose of replacement hormone is changed until the TSH is normal. However, if the cause is central hypothyroidism, the TSH cannot be used as a guide because the pituitary is not making any TSH.

In some cases, starting the child at a low dose and gradually increasing to the full therapeutic dose may be necessary. Some children show more symptoms when they suddenly go from no thyroid hormone to full replacement. They experience trouble sleeping, restlessness, and deterioration in their school performance. A rare patient will have headaches due to increased pressure in the brain. Lowering the dose and gradually building it back up will manage this situation.

If the child's growth has been delayed, he or she usually catches up when thyroid hormone is given.

Giving too much thyroid hormone may cause early bone closure resulting in stunted growth and a decrease in the mineral content of the bone.

Dealing with Hyperthyroidism in Children

Hyperthyroidism is rarely seen in babies and is less common in children and adolescents than it is in adults. Almost always, kids with hyperthyroidism have Graves' disease (see Chapter 6). When a newborn is hyperthyroid, usually the mother is also hyperthyroid (see Chapter 16), and the mother's thyroid-stimulating antibodies have been passed to the fetus. When these antibodies are cleared from the fetus after it is born, the hyperthyroidism subsides about 3 to 12 weeks after birth.

Signs and symptoms

When the mother with hyperthyroidism passes a large amount of thyroid-stimulating antibodies to the fetus through the placenta, the fetus develops hyperthyroidism. The signs of the hyperthyroidism in the fetus include:

✔ Rapid heart rate

✔ Increased fetal movements

✔ Poor fetal body growth

✔ Abnormally rapid bone growth

After the baby is born, the baby shows a number of signs and symptoms of hyperthyroidism. They are the result of excessive metabolism in a baby who should be growing and developing normally. These signs and symptoms include:

✔ Low birth weight and failure to gain weight

✔ Increased appetite

✔ Irritability

✔ Rapid heart rate

✔ Enlarged thyroid

✔ Prominent eyes

Hyperthyroidism is rare in children under the age of 5 and is usually caused by Graves' disease. Once in a while, the cause may be a functioning thyroid adenoma, a new growth of tissue on or within the thyroid that is making excessive amounts of thyroid hormone. Girls are more often affected than boys by thyroid adenomas. A family history of other autoimmune diseases may be found if the cause is Graves' disease.

In children under the age of 5, the signs and symptoms of hyperthyroidism are like those seen in adults (see Chapter 6), again tempered by the needs of a growing child who has now reached school age. Unique signs at this age include the following:

- ✔ Poor school performance
- ✔ Trouble sleeping
- ✔ Poor athletic performance related to muscle weakness
- ✔ Tiredness
- ✔ More rapid growth in height but early closure of bone growth
- ✔ Irritability

These children are hungry all the time but don't gain weight despite eating. They generally have mild eye disease. They have goiters and also have bowel movements more frequently than they should.

Laboratory confirmation

Confirmation of the diagnosis of hyperthyroidism is accomplished by obtaining a free T4 and a TSH level. If fetal hyperthyroidism is suspected, these levels can be determined from umbilical-cord blood at birth. If hyperthyroidism is present, the free T4 will be high and the TSH low. Rarely, if the hyperthyroidism is due to excessive TSH secretion from the pituitary, the TSH will be high. In that case, the doctor should be on the lookout for a pituitary tumor.

Treatment

If your child has hyperthyroidism, you have many treatment options. The important thing to remember is that your scrutiny does not end with treatment, because all forms of treatment can be associated with the recurrence of hyperthyroidism or the development of hypothyroidism.

Be sure that your child's condition is followed up regularly after treatment because the disease process is ongoing. Regularly means every six months or yearly, as recommended by your doctor.

If the fetus is hyperthyroid, antithyroid drugs are given to the mother. The drugs pass through the placenta to affect the fetus's thyroid hormone production. The goal is to have a fetal heart rate less than 140 beats per minute. Sometimes, the mother takes a beta blocker (such as propranolol) to control severe symptoms.

Treatment of hyperthyroidism in babies is also done with antithyroid drugs. Once treatment is given, the baby rapidly improves. In a few months, the antithyroid drugs are withdrawn because the thyroid-stimulating antibodies that were passed from mother to baby disappear from the baby.

Radioactive iodine

At one time, doctors resisted using radioactive iodine to treat hyperthyroidism in children. However, this treatment is commonly used today because long-term studies have shown no negative effects upon the child. Specifically, there's no increase in cancer or loss of fertility and no negative effect upon the offspring of children treated with radioactive iodine.

The problem with radioactive iodine is that most children become hypothyroid after some time. (The same is true of adults; see Chapter 6.) In addition, thyroid eye disease may get worse when radioactive iodine is used because of the release of a lot of antigen from the thyroid.

Antithyroid drugs

Antithyroid drugs such as propylthiouricil (PTU) and methimazole are the preferred treatment for hyperthyroidism in children. They take 3 to 6 weeks to work, but they control the disease in at least 85 percent of children. If the medication doesn't work, the child either has a very large goiter or doesn't take the medication as prescribed. In most cases, the treatment is continued for 2 to 4 years.

How does the doctor choose which of these drugs to use? PTU has the advantage of blocking the conversion of T4 to T3, whereas methimazole lasts longer after taking it. In practice, these differences don't seem to matter much. I tend to use methimazole only because I have more experience with it, not because I believe it's better.

If the disease is going to recur after the pills are stopped, the child usually has measurable amounts of TSH receptor-stimulating antibodies. This test is done at the time treatment is stopped to help to predict a recurrence. The drugs may fail to produce a permanent remission in up to half the patients treated, even though 85 percent can be controlled.

Just as in adults, antithyroid medications cause side effects in children. The most important is that the production of white blood cells can be halted. The doctor should monitor white blood cells, and if the white cell count is less than 1,000, the drug must be stopped. If PTU was used initially, the child is not switched to methimazole and vice versa. A totally different treatment is given. Sometimes, the white cell count falls a little, but it returns to normal after some weeks. Another important side effect is the development of a rash, which can be treated without needing to stop taking the drug.

Surgery of the thyroid

Sometimes, antithyroid drugs cause serious side effects or the child doesn't take the pills correctly, and radioactive iodine can't be used (usually because the parents are concerned about giving radioactivity to their child). In these cases, surgery is a safe and rapid form of treatment when done by a competent surgeon who has experience with children. If possible, the child should have normal thyroid function accomplished with the antithyroid drugs before going to surgery. Iodine is given for two weeks prior to surgery to block the thyroid gland and reduce blood flow into it. The usual operation is a near total thyroidectomy (see Chapter 13).

It may be possible to leave enough thyroid tissue to retain thyroid function while eliminating hyperthyroidism, but the child must be checked at least every six months to a year to detect recurrence or loss of thyroid function and the need for thyroid medication.

Diagnosing Goiters in Children

An enlarged thyroid gland is actually the most common thyroid abnormality found in children. It occurs in about 5 percent of all children. A child with an enlarged thyroid usually has normal thyroid function.

The most common cause of thyroid enlargement in children is autoimmune thyroiditis (see Chapter 5). The second most common cause is a multinodular goiter (see Chapter 9).

Differentiating between these causes is important because autoimmune thyroiditis can lead to hypothyroidism (or sometimes hyperthyroidism), whereas multinodular goiter does not. Obtaining thyroid autoantibody studies will tell the difference, pointing to autoimmune thyroiditis if the results are positive. Testing the child's levels of free T4 and TSH will verify that his or her thyroid function is normal.

These goiters sometimes get smaller and then larger again, sometimes growing at different rates in different parts of the thyroid, leading to a multinodular thyroid gland.

Treatment is given if the large thyroid is pressing on nearby structures like the esophagus and trachea or is disfiguring. The treatment will be either surgery or radioactive iodine. The thyroid is checked every six months for a few visits, then yearly.

If the goiter is painful, the diagnosis is more likely subacute or acute thyroiditis (see Chapter 11). These diseases cause similar signs and symptoms in children as they cause in adults. Subacute thyroiditis generally makes a child less sick than does acute thyroiditis. Subacute thyroiditis affects the whole gland, whereas acute thyroiditis may swell only part of the gland. If acute thyroiditis occurs several times, there may be a malformation in the thyroid that will probably require surgery.

Nodules and Cancer in Children

Children rarely get thyroid nodules, but when they do, the nodules indicate cancer more frequently than they do in adults. The signs that make a nodule particularly suspicious for cancer are the same as in adults: rapid growth, painlessness, firmness and fixation, and nodes felt in the neck. While a functioning nodule or a cystic nodule (see Chapter 7) is rarely found to be cancer in an adult, this isn't true in children.

A very important clue that a child's nodule may be cancerous is past exposure to irradiation. Exposure leads to nodules and cancer in multiple places in the thyroid. (The leading type of thyroid cancer in both children and adults is *papillary* — the type of cancer most closely associated with irradiation exposure.) Exposure to X-rays is not limited to people living in the area around a nuclear power plant. In the United States, in the not-so-distant past, X-rays were used to treat acne and enlarged thymus glands (which lie near the thyroid).

A fine needle biopsy of the nodule is done if the doctor suspects cancer, but this test isn't as helpful in children as it is in adults. A 1996 study in the *Journal of Pediatric Surgery* showed that a correct diagnosis of thyroid cancer was made in only 3 of 7 biopsies. It's not clear why this is so — perhaps because the child's nodule is small and easily missed by the needle.

Children tend to have more cancer spread in the neck and into the lungs at the time they are diagnosed than adults do, but this does not make their prognosis worse. The cancer can be managed just like adult cancer with a total thyroidectomy (see Chapter 13), preserving the parathyroid glands and the recurrent laryngeal nerves. This is followed by radioactive ablation of the remaining thyroid tissue. The patient is placed on thyroid hormone to replace the thyroid and to suppress growth of new thyroid tissue.

Children with thyroid cancer are monitored with thyroglobulin blood tests; this test should read close to 0 shortly after surgery. The blood tests are done every 6 months to a year. If the level of thyroglobulin rises, a whole body scan is done looking for tissue that takes up iodine. The scan can be done using the new recombinant TSH (see Chapter 15) so the patient does not have to stop taking thyroid hormone to perform this study. If all the iodine is found in the neck, local surgery may be enough to eliminate the additional thyroid cancer tissue. If the tissue is spread around the body, a large dose of radioactive iodine will destroy it.

Chapter 18

Thyroid Disease and the Elderly

*B*efore we start talking thyroids, let's get our definitions straight. Who is "elderly"? The answer to this question becomes more and more important to me as I get older. For the sake of the information in this chapter, let's accept the definition used in most studies, namely, a person age 65 or older.

Elderly people are often afflicted with thyroid disease. The trouble with thyroid disease in the elderly, and the reason that I devote an entire chapter to it, is that it's so often missed. It's missed for two key reasons. First, when an elderly person goes to a doctor, hospital, or nursing home, the illness or condition that prompts her to seek care is, naturally, the doctor's primary focus. Second, symptoms of thyroid disease often mirror symptoms of other conditions, so even if the doctor looks for other conditions in the patient, thyroid disease in the elderly is easily misdiagnosed.

When doctors are taught about disease, they learn a set of signs and symptoms that are characteristic of the disease. Elderly patients with thyroid disease may have none of the symptoms typical of the disease, or their symptoms may be almost opposite of what we expect. The only way doctors are going to discover thyroid disease in many elderly patients is with screening — obtaining thyroid function tests from a person who appears to be healthy.

Screening for thyroid disease in the elderly has its own problems. The main problem is that screening picks up a lot of *subclinical disease* — a situation where one blood test is not normal but another is, and the patient has no symptoms of the disease. There's tremendous controversy concerning what to do with subclinical thyroid disease. As a community, doctors haven't yet made any final decisions about whether to treat subclinical thyroid disease, wait for symptoms to develop, or wait for both thyroid blood tests to become abnormal. In this chapter, I share my own biases as I discuss the various diseases.

The Extent of the Problem

To determine how many elderly people are affected by thyroid disease, we need yet another definition. How do we define "thyroid disease"? Is it sufficient to have an abnormal TSH level to make a diagnosis, or must the free T4 level be abnormal as well? (See Chapter 4 for information about these tests.) This is difficult to answer in the elderly because they often have so many symptoms; many of these are symptoms of other conditions, as well as thyroid disease.

Some doctors consider an abnormal TSH to be insufficient evidence of thyroid disease; they use the term *subclinical* to describe the situation where the TSH is abnormal but the free T4 is normal. They advocate against treating a patient with subclinical thyroid disease. Yet many studies have shown that treatment reduces or eliminates many of the symptoms. On the other hand, treating an elderly person, particularly with thyroid hormone for hypothyroidism, may not be entirely benign and helpful, as I discuss later in this chapter.

In one study from the United Kingdom, published in the *Archives of Internal Medicine* in January 2001, all patients age 65 or older were tested for thyroid disease when they entered the hospital. Out of 280 patients (leaving out those who already were known to have thyroid disease), 9 had hypothyroidism and 5 had hyperthyroidism. None of these 14 cases had previously been suspected. An additional 21 patients had subclinical hypothyroidism (high TSH, normal free T4), and 12 had subclinical hyperthyroidism (low TSH, normal free T4). The authors stated that overall, nearly 40 percent of the elderly people not thought to have thyroid disease had some evidence of it. Should all these people receive some treatment?

Writing in rebuttal to this study, other authors suggested that many of the people with subclinical disease are actually found to have temporary abnormalities caused by other diseases.

In another study of elderly people who were not hospitalized, unsuspected hyperthyroidism was discovered in 1 percent, and unsuspected hypothyroidism was discovered in 2 percent. So, 3 of 100 elderly people are walking around with clinical thyroid disease. That may not seem like a lot, but in the population of the United States, it means that there are almost one million elderly people walking around with undetected and highly treatable thyroid disease. (That number does not even account for the age group 35 to 65, which contains many more cases of undiagnosed thyroid disease.)

Large population studies have shown that 10 percent of women over age 65 have elevated TSH levels. Most of them do not have symptoms of thyroid disease.

I find it interesting that there's no argument about screening babies for thyroid disease (when the occurrence of abnormal tests is 1 in 3,750), yet the debate continues about screening the elderly (when 3 in 100 cases of clinical thyroid disease may be found).

My own bias is that everyone should be screened for thyroid disease beginning at age 35 and every 5 years thereafter. Screening is easily done with a TSH test. If this test is abnormal, then a free T4 test is done. If both tests are abnormal, the patient is treated for thyroid disease. If only the TSH is abnormal, it's reasonable to take a careful history and do a physical examination, and then decide on treatment based upon that evaluation. Other factors can be taken into consideration when making the decision whether to treat; later in the chapter, I discuss these factors in relation to specific diseases.

Sources of Confusion in Diagnosis

The natural consequences of aging, the many complicating diseases found in the elderly, and medications can all confuse a diagnosis of thyroid disease. Aging and other diseases can cause symptoms that may be identical to those found in thyroid disease. Medications cause changes in laboratory tests that confuse the diagnosis (see Chapter 10).

Other diseases

Certain diseases that are found more often in the elderly than in younger people cause changes in thyroid function test results, which make it appear as though the patient has thyroid disease. The more common conditions and diseases that confuse thyroid testing are

- Poor nutrition
- Poorly controlled diabetes mellitus
- Liver disease
- Heart failure

Severe illness causes a temporary fall in T4 that may be misdiagnosed as hypothyroidism.

Medications

Drugs often taken by the elderly that can alter thyroid function tests include the following:

- ✔ Epilepsy drugs such as carbamazine and diphenylhydantoin cause the rapid breakdown of thyroid hormones by the liver, which lowers thyroid hormone levels in the blood.

- ✔ Aspirin decreases the binding of thyroid hormones to thyroid-binding globulin, thereby lowering the total (but not the free) T4.

- ✔ Arthritis drugs such as prednisone decrease thyroxine binding globulin levels.

- ✔ Drugs for abnormal heart rhythm, particularly amiodarone, can cause both hypothyroidism and hyperthyroidism.

- ✔ Heparin, used for anticoagulation, can cause a temporary rise in T4 by displacing it from binding proteins.

Discovering Hypothyroidism in the Elderly

Victor Brooklyn is a 68-year-old man who has been feeling a bit fatigued lately. He has put on a few pounds, and he feels cold when others seem comfortable. He also notices that he is more constipated than before. Victor thinks that all these changes are the natural effects of aging. He had been constipated for years, but it has recently become a serious problem, and this is what brings him to his doctor. The doctor observes that Victor's pulse is slow and that he has lost some of his eyelashes. He tells Victor that he believes this may be hypothyroidism and sends him for thyroid function tests.

The TSH level comes back high at 9, but the free T4 is within the normal range. Because his doctor is unsure of what to do, he sends Victor to Dr. Rubin. Dr. Rubin tells Victor that he appears to have subclinical hypothyroidism, although he thinks that the symptoms that Victor describes are being caused by his thyroid. He puts Victor on thyroid hormone replacement pills.

After two weeks, Victor notices that his bowel movements have improved. He is less tired and less cold. He returns to Dr. Rubin for repeat thyroid function tests. The TSH is now 6, so Dr. Rubin increases the dose of thyroid hormone. A month later, the TSH test is down in the normal range, and Victor states that he is now just his mildly constipated self.

Deciphering signs and symptoms

The diagnosis of hypothyroidism is so easily missed in the elderly that I have to admit I have missed it myself on occasion (very rare occasions, of course). The principal reason is that so many of the changes our bodies experience as we grow older are typical findings in hypothyroidism. Some of the most important are the following:

- Slowing of mental function
- Slowing of physical function
- Tendency to have a lower body temperature
- Intolerance of cold
- Constipation
- Hardening of the arteries
- Elevation of blood fats (especially cholesterol)
- Weight gain
- Elevation of blood pressure
- Anemia
- Muscle cramps
- Dry skin

All the above changes are common effects of aging but are also signs and symptoms of hypothyroidism.

On the other hand, some signs found in the elderly would tend to point away from a diagnosis of hypothyroidism, making an accurate diagnosis even less likely. For example, the elderly get Parkinson's disease, which results in tremors, or they simply develop senile tremors. Many elderly people lose weight because of poor nutrition; they may also be nervous. These symptoms may point to an overactive thyroid, but they definitely don't neatly fit into the list of symptoms of hypothyroidism.

Many elderly person with hypothyroidism do not have goiters.

Getting laboratory confirmation

The only way to know for sure that an elderly person does not have hypothyroidism is to obtain thyroid function tests. If hypothyroidism is present, the free T4 should be low and the TSH should be high (see Chapter 4). Often the TSH is high but the free T4 is normal — the situation known as *subclinical hypothyroidism.* The only way to determine whether hypothyroidism is having an effect upon the patient is to give a trial of thyroid hormone. I am very much in favor of doing this although, as I explain in the next section, the patient may not feel much different on medication.

Trying thyroid hormone for subclinical patients

Among elderly patients with subclinical thyroid disease whose TSH level is less than 10, only half show some clinical improvement after receiving thyroxine (T4 hormone replacement). Such patients should probably not be treated if they complain of anginal heart pain. Every patient whose TSH level is over 20 will improve with treatment.

An important study, whose results indicate that subclinical hypothyroidism in the elderly should be treated, was published in *Clinical Endocrinology* in 2000. It was a study of 1,843 people ages 55 and over. All were evaluated for the presence of hypothyroidism. Of those individuals in the study who had an elevated TSH but a normal free T4, the risk of dementia and Alzheimer's disease was three times greater than those with normal TSH and free T4 when the patients were followed for as short a time as just two years. The lower the free T4 (though still in the normal range), the higher the incidence of dementia and Alzheimer's. Those individuals who had positive antiperoxidase antibodies (see Chapter 4) also had a higher incidence of dementia. The authors' conclusion was, "This is the first prospective study to suggest that subclinical hypothyroidism in the elderly increases the risk of dementia and Alzheimer's disease."

Another factor that influences treatment decisions is that an elderly patient who has subclinical hypothyroidism along with another autoimmune disorder — such as type 1 diabetes, pernicious anemia, rheumatoid arthritis, or premature graying of the hair — is likely to eventually become clinically hypothyroid.

If you have subclinical thyroid disease and your doctor starts you on thyroid hormone replacement, there are several reasons why you may want to continue that treatment. If you test positive for thyroid autoantibodies and you have a high TSH, chances are very good that you'll develop clinical hypothyroidism in the future. Also, your cholesterol level may benefit from the thyroid hormone; a measurement of cholesterol before and after taking the pills may show that it has been lowered significantly. A chemical in the blood called *homocysteine,* which can contribute to heart disease, is also often lowered by the thyroid hormone.

Taking treatment slowly

As far as treatment is concerned, it's most important that the doctor go slowly. He or she should start with a very low dose of thyroxine (for example, 25 micrograms), increasing it every 4 to 6 weeks until the TSH is at the upper limit of normal. You do not want excessive treatment because it can possibly worsen heart pain and increase shortness of breath, palpitations, and rapid heartbeats, as well as nervousness and heat intolerance. Even the first exposure to a small dose of thyroxine may bring on anginal chest pain. A dose that is excessive causes osteoporosis, a thinning of the bones.

The major problem doctors have when treating elderly patients with hypothyroidism may be one of compliance — ensuring that a patient is taking his or her medication. If you have a parent in this situation, putting the pills into a case with daily slots may help. Ultimately, only someone standing there, observing the drug being taken, can be sure.

It's important to test thyroid function on a regular basis to ensure that the TSH and free T4 levels remain normal. Testing every six months should be adequate.

Hyperthyroidism in the Elderly

Toby Dummy is the 76-year-old aunt of Stacy and Karen Dummy. Her husband has noticed that she seems depressed lately. While she used to love to cook, she seems to have lost interest. She sits on her couch most of the day, not doing much of anything. She has gained several pounds and seems fatigued most of the time. Toby's doctor suggests that perhaps she is hypothyroid. He obtains thyroid function tests. To his surprise, the free T4 is elevated and the TSH is suppressed, suggesting a diagnosis of hyperthyroidism. He sends Toby to see Dr. Rubin.

Dr. Rubin, whose practice is filled with members of the Dummy family by this time, examines Toby and finds that she does not have a goiter. However, her pulse is somewhat fast. He makes a diagnosis of *apathetic hyperthyroidism* and explains to Toby's husband that this type of hyperthyroidism is not uncommon in the elderly population. He starts Toby on the antithyroid drug methimazole. After six weeks, Toby's thyroid function tests are normal. The methimazole is stopped and Toby is given radioactive iodine several days later.

Toby is feeling so much better that she invites Dr. Rubin and his wife, Enid, to a delicious dinner in a lovely dining room recently remodeled by Toby's husband.

Sorting through confusing signs and symptoms

Hyperthyroidism is less common than hypothyroidism, but it's still a significant problem among the elderly. As with hypothyroidism, the symptoms of an overactive thyroid can be easily confused with the normal signs of aging. The following characteristics are among the similarities between normal aging and hyperthyroidism:

✔ The patients often shake.

✔ They lose weight.

✔ They have irregular heart rhythms.

✔ Congestive heart failure is an increased threat.

✔ Patients have intolerance to heat.

✔ They sweat a lot.

✔ They experience fatigue and weakness.

At the same time, the elderly may have signs that are not consistent with hyperthyroidism at all. They may appear entirely apathetic, sitting very quietly, acting depressed, and showing fatigue and weight gain. This is the picture of apathetic hyperthyroidism illustrated by Toby Dummy.

Many elderly patients with hyperthyroidism do not have goiters.

Sometimes the first sign of hyperthyroidism is the finding of *atrial fibrillation,* an irregular heartbeat. (If you're diagnosed with atrial fibrillation, you may need to take an anticoagulant to prevent *pulmonary emboli,* blood clots that form in the irregularly beating heart and flow to the lungs, cutting off blood flow when they become stuck. After the heart rhythm is restored to normal, the anticoagulant can be stopped.)

If your heart rhythm has suddenly become very irregular, and your doctor tells you that it's atrial fibrillation, ask him or her to order thyroid function tests.

Loss of bone is another important consequence of hyperthyroidism. The elderly, particularly women who already have much diminished bone, cannot afford to lose more bone. One study, published in the *Journal of Clinical Investigation* in 2000, showed that elderly people with hyperthyroidism had significant reduction in bone density when compared with elderly people without hyperthyroidism. After hyperthyroid patients were successfully treated, their bone mineral density showed improvement within six months. Other studies have shown that there's a definite increase in bone fracture risk in people with hyperthyroidism.

Securing a diagnosis

Thyroid function tests remain the key method for making a diagnosis of hyperthyroidism in the elderly. If hyperthyroidism is present, the free T4 should be high and the TSH should be suppressed. Occasionally, the T4 is normal but the free T3 is elevated, a condition called *T3 thyrotoxicosis* (see Chapter 6). This condition is especially common if a hyperactive nodule is the source of the hyperthyroidism.

The treatment of choice for hyperthyroidism in the elderly is *radioactive iodine* (RAI). With a single treatment, the disease is brought under control in four to six weeks. RAI avoids the problems associated with taking the daily antithyroid pills. However, many people who take RAI develop hypothyroidism and need to be on a daily thyroid hormone pill for the rest of their lives.

A beta blocker such as propranolol is also useful in controlling symptoms of hyperthyroidism (such as tremor, nervousness, sweating, and rapid heart rate).

If RAI is given to a hyperactive thyroid, there may be a sudden release of thyroid hormones as the thyroid tissues break down. This may be dangerous for an elderly person, who could have a sudden worsening of heart failure and a very rapid heart rate, as well as much worse chest pain. To avoid this complication, antithyroid drugs are given for six weeks before the RAI is administered. When the patient has normal thyroid function on the drugs, the risk of a sudden release of thyroid hormones is eliminated.

Most heart symptoms associated with hyperthyroidism disappear after treatment is successful. However, sometimes the atrial fibrillation does not reverse.

Thyroid Nodules in the Elderly

Nodules are very common in the elderly, but thyroid cancer is found less often in elderly people than in younger people. The nodules can be studied with a radioactive iodine scan to see whether they are active and an ultrasound to see whether they are filled with fluid *(cystic)*. Both of these characteristics point the diagnosis to a benign nodule rather than a cancer. Thyroid function tests can show whether the nodule is hyperfunctioning and needs to be treated.

In the final analysis, a fine needle aspiration biopsy remains the best single test to rule out cancer in a nodule. Should this test be positive for cancer, surgery is the treatment of choice, with follow-up similar to any thyroid cancer patient (see Chapter 8).

Chapter 19

Diet, Exercise, and Your Thyroid

*E*ven after all these chapters, you probably have some important lingering questions about your thyroid. This chapter can answer them and offer further evidence (in case you still need it) of the starring role that the thyroid gland plays in your body.

Remember that your thyroid gland functions at its best if it finds itself in a healthy body whose tissues have been fed by the right nutrients and whose muscles and bones have been strengthened by an appropriate level of exercise. For this reason, I give you some basic ideas about diet and exercise here. For a more complete guide to diet, see my book *Diabetes Cookbook For Dummies,* which contains dietary suggestions not just for people with diabetes, but for all people who want to eat healthy food. To learn more about exercise in your lifestyle, see *Diabetes For Dummies,* which presents an exercise program for anyone who wants to feel good in his or her body. Both these titles are published by Hungry Minds, Inc.

Guaranteeing Your Best Nutrition

Two friends run into each other, and the first friend asks how the second one feels. The second friend answers, "Lousy, I've got arthritis, a bad back, I'm always tense, I have insomnia. Miserable, I'm miserable." "And what kind of work are you doing?" the first friend asks. "The same thing — I'm still selling health foods."

This story is good for a chuckle, but the truth is that what you eat (and drink and smoke) has more influence on your health than all the diseases in a textbook of medicine.

In the United States, we spend more than $100 billion on health each year. (That goes a long way toward explaining all the healthy doctors in this country.)

The U.S. government is very aware of all these health costs and knows that its citizens function best when they eat right and exercise. For this reason, the government has long published a list of recommendations called the "Dietary Guidelines for Americans." These guidelines are a great place for you to start to turn your body into a suitable "container" for a healthy thyroid gland. In the year 2000 edition, the guidelines are clustered into three groups:

✔ Aim for fitness.

- Aim for a healthy weight.

- Be physically active each day.

✔ Build a healthy base.

- Choose a variety of grains daily, especially whole grains.

- Choose a variety of fruits and vegetables daily.

- Keep food safe to eat.

✔ Choose sensibly.

- Choose beverages and foods to moderate your intake of sugars.

- Choose and prepare foods with less salt.

- If you drink alcoholic beverages, do so in moderation.

The following section gets more specific about these recommendations.

Maintaining a healthy weight

If you go online and check out a message board about thyroid disease, you'll probably find that lots of people have lots of questions about how the thyroid affects weight gain and loss. This section helps set the record straight.

There's a very simple way to determine your ideal weight; the calculation differs slightly for men and women. The key is your height.

If you are a man, calculate your height in inches. Give yourself 106 pounds for the first 60 inches (5 feet) of height, and 6 pounds for each inch above 60. For example, a 5'6" man should weight 106 plus 6 times 6, or 142 pounds. This would be his ideal weight. However, there really is a weight *range* that is appropriate for each height, because each of us has a different body shape. To calculate the range, take 10 percent of the number you calculate as your ideal weight, and add that number to and subtract it from the ideal weight number. For example, the man who is 5'6" would determine that 10 percent of 142 is 14 pounds. He'd add 14 to 142 and subtract 14 from 142 to get his weight range. The range for a 5'6" man would be 128 to 156 pounds.

For a woman, calculate your height in inches and give yourself 100 pounds for the first 60 inches (5 feet), then 5 pounds for each inch over 60. A 5'4" woman has an ideal weight of 120 pounds. Using the same technique described in the previous paragraph, she would calculate that her proper weight range is 108 to 132 pounds.

Now that you know how much you should weigh, how can you achieve that goal? This is where we can use the government's helpful suggestions.

Using the Food Guide Pyramid to make your food choices

The Food Guide Pyramid looks a lot like the pyramids in Egypt. The base of the pyramid consists of the foods that you eat the most of in a day, and the pyramid narrows up to the foods with the highest calories and least nutrition, which you should eat sparingly. It includes all the foods that you can possibly eat:

- Breads, cereals, rice, and pasta create the base of the pyramid. You may have 6 to 11 servings of these foods daily.

- Fruits and vegetables are the second level of the pyramid. You may have 2 to 4 servings of fruit and 3 to 5 servings of vegetables each day.

- Two categories of food combine to form the third level of the pyramid. You may have 2 to 3 servings of meat, poultry, fish, dry beans, eggs, and nuts each day. You may also have 2 to 3 servings from the milk, yogurt, and cheese group.

- The top level of the pyramid contains the fats, oils, and sweets — foods that are to be used sparingly.

The first question that you want answered is probably "What is a serving?" Although space does not allow me to list every possible food and what constitutes a serving for that food, here is a general guide to serving size:

- **Bread, cereal, rice, and pasta:** A serving is one slice of bread; 1 ounce of ready-to-eat cereal; or ½ cup of cooked cereal, rice, or pasta.

✔ **Fruit:** A serving is one medium apple, banana, or orange; ½ cup of chopped, cooked, or canned fruit; or ¾ cup of fruit juice.

✔ **Vegetables:** A serving is 1 cup of raw leafy vegetables; ½ cup of other vegetables, cooked or chopped raw; or ¾ cup of vegetable juice.

✔ **Meat, poultry, fish, dry beans, eggs, or nuts:** A serving is 2 to 3 ounces of cooked lean meat, poultry, or fish; ½ cup of cooked dry beans; or 1 egg. Two tablespoons of peanut butter count as 1 ounce of meat.

✔ **Milk, yogurt, and cheese:** A serving is 1 cup of milk or yogurt, 1½ ounces of natural cheese, or 2 ounces of processed cheese.

You can find serving sizes for all foods in the U.S. government publication "Dietary Guidelines for Americans."

Counting calories

The guidelines explained in the previous section offer a range of servings of each food group rather than a fixed number of servings. The reason for this is that your number of daily servings depends on your ideal weight. Also, because no two people are exactly alike in their metabolism and in their activity level, a daily calorie level for two people of the same height and weight will be different, particularly if they are male and female. But you can get a general idea of how many calories you should be consuming to maintain your ideal weight, and then make adjustments if you find that you need fewer or more calories.

Start with the figure for your ideal weight (see the previous section "Maintaining a healthy weight"). Multiply that number by 10. If you should weigh 140 pounds, for example, your calculation comes to 1,400 kilocalories, which is your basal calorie need. Now you add more depending on your activity level. A person who does not exercise much at all will increase the basal calorie number by 10 percent, to give a daily kilocalorie level of 1,540. A person who does moderate exercise, for example a daily walk for 25 minutes, would add 20 percent to that total to give 1,680 kilocalories. The very active person, who digs ditches all day for example, would need 40 percent more or even higher to give a daily need of 1,960 kilocalories or greater.

How do you translate daily calories into daily servings? Because the calorie content of the servings is known, you can create a daily diet by adding up the calories in the servings in the Food Guide Pyramid, keeping the number of servings for each food group at the recommended level. In Table 19-1, the U.S. government has done some groundwork for you.

Table 19-1	Recommended Servings to Meet Calorie Needs		
Food Group	*1,600 Kilocalories*	*2,200 Kilocalories*	*2,800 Kilocalories*
Bread, cereal, rice, and pasta	6 servings	9 servings	11 servings
Vegetables	3 servings	4 servings	5 servings
Fruits	2 servings	3 servings	4 servings
Milk, yogurt, and cheese	3 servings	3 servings	3 servings
Meats, poultry, fish, dry beans, eggs, and nuts	2 servings (total 5 ounces)	2 servings (total 6 ounces)	3 servings (total 7 ounces)

If you adhere to these guidelines, you are well on your way to hitting the target of a healthy weight. The next sections fine-tune this information by discussing individual nutrients and why you ought to choose a variety of grains, fruits, and vegetables.

Selecting a variety of foods

Choosing among the many foods that make up each group has many benefits. Most important, when you eat a variety of foods, you ensure that you get all the nutrients needed by your body (including your thyroid). In particular, some foods contain certain vitamins and minerals that are not present in other foods. Only a variety of foods will get you all the vitamins and minerals that you need. In addition, your meals are more interesting when you eat a variety of foods rather than the same meal again and again.

Keep in mind that despite their differences in color and appearance, most fruits and vegetables share about the same energy sources as other members of their group (see the following section). The different colors and appearances indicate that they differ in their vitamins and minerals.

Energy sources

The energy that we use to move our bodies comes from one of three sources: protein, carbohydrate, or fat. Protein is necessary to build muscles and the organs of the body. Proteins also make up certain hormones. The backbone of the thyroid hormone is an amino acid, one of the several amino acids that combine to make up protein.

You get your protein when you eat animal foods such as meat, fish, poultry, and milk. These are sources of complete protein. Each of these foods contains all the amino acids that the human body needs to manufacture its own protein, including certain amino acids that the human body cannot manufacture called *essential amino acids*. Plants, especially beans and peas, also contain protein, but a single source of vegetable protein does not have all the essential amino acids in one food source. Therefore, vegetarians must eat a variety of protein sources.

Carbohydrates are mainly found in the bread, cereal, rice, and pasta food group, as well as in fruits and some vegetables. When carbohydrates are broken down in the intestine, they are absorbed into the body as sugars, which give you the immediate energy that you need to move your muscles. They can also be stored in your muscles and your liver to provide energy if you need it later on.

Fats are needed in very small quantities to provide the backbone for certain essential hormones such as estrogen and testosterone. They also store energy in the fat tissues of your body, but when they are present in excessive amounts, they can accumulate in places where they do damage, especially the arteries of the heart. The worst offenders are the saturated fats, the kind that are solid at room temperature. Butter and the fat attached to a steak are examples. The calories in this type of fat should make up no more than 10 percent of your total calories. Most of the fats of vegetable origin (like canola oil and olive oil) are not saturated fats, although they are still a source of concentrated calories. Vegetable fats that are saturated are coconut and palm oils, which should be used sparingly.

Vitamins

Vitamins are needed in tiny amounts but are essential for a healthy body. They are used to change the stored energy in the energy sources into energy that can be used by the body. They are used in many of the chemical reactions that take place in the cells of your body. There are a number of vitamins that you need to eat because your body cannot make them. The various vitamins, their function, and their sources in food include the following:

- Vitamin A, used for vision and growth of bone and teeth, is found in liver, carrots, and spinach.
- Vitamin B1, used for digestion and nervous system function, comes from whole-grain cereals, peas, and nuts.
- Vitamin B2, which helps to release energy and maintain the skin and eyes, comes from liver, milk, eggs, and leafy vegetables.
- Vitamin B3, used for maintenance of the skin and nerves, comes from chicken, salmon, and peanuts.

✔ Vitamin B6 is needed to make red blood cells and to release energy from the energy sources. It comes from meat, fish, poultry, and peanuts.

✔ Vitamin B12 is essential for the nervous system and red blood cells. It's found in all foods coming from animals, including meat and milk; a person who eats nothing but vegetables will not get this vitamin.

✔ Vitamin C helps with healing and prevention of infections and is found in citrus fruits, strawberries, and broccoli.

✔ Vitamin D is required for the proper use of calcium and comes in milk, fish, and the yolk of eggs. Fortunately, this is a vitamin that can be made by the body when the skin is exposed to sunlight.

✔ Vitamin E has many functions including prevention of cholesterol buildup and production of red blood cells and muscles. You get it in vegetable oils, peas, and nuts.

✔ Vitamin K is essential for clotting of the blood so that you don't continue to bleed when you are cut. It comes in broccoli and leafy vegetables.

✔ Folic acid is another vitamin needed to produce red blood cells and protein. It's found in leafy vegetables, oranges, and peanuts.

Minerals

The minerals are not *organic* — that means they are not of animal or vegetable origin. They come from the earth and are taken up by vegetables, which are then eaten by animals. Minerals consist of the major minerals, which are present in relatively large amounts in the body, and trace elements that are essential but present in only tiny amounts.

The major minerals consist of the following:

✔ Calcium for strong bones and teeth, for blood clotting, and for muscle function is found in dairy products, almonds, broccoli and other green vegetables.

✔ Magnesium for nerve and muscle function is found in milk, seafood, bananas, and green leafy vegetables.

✔ Phosphorus for the bones and teeth comes from milk, hamburger, and cheese.

The trace elements include:

✔ Chromium for using carbohydrates properly, which is found in organ meats, mushrooms, and broccoli.

✔ Iodine, the key mineral for the production of thyroid hormones, which is found in seafood and iodized salt and bread.

✔ Iron for red blood cell hemoglobin, which comes from meat, poultry, fish, and raisins.

✔ Selenium, also used in enzymes that affect thyroid hormones, which is found in seafood and whole grains.

✔ Zinc, needed in the production of insulin and found in red meat, shellfish, and eggs.

Now you know what these nutrients are, what they do, and where they can be found. No discussion of proper nutrition could leave out a discussion of fats, so keep reading.

Choosing your fats properly

You want to limit your fat intake to no more than 30 percent of your total daily calories while limiting your intake of saturated fat to no more than one third of that amount. Eating your calories according to the Food Guide Pyramid will keep you within those limitations if you choose your fats wisely. Select foods that contain unsaturated fat, like vegetable oils (not coconut or palm oils).

You can keep your fats down by looking for low-fat foods, which are plentiful in the supermarkets these days. Just remember not to substitute foods rich in carbohydrates. Food labels can tell you what you need to know about the energy sources in the food as well as the amounts of the vitamins and minerals.

The fat that most people think about is cholesterol. You should know your level of cholesterol. Ask your doctor to check your cholesterol level if you don't know it yet. The recommendation is that your total cholesterol should be less than 200. However, there is a particle in your blood called *high density lipoprotein* (HDL) that carries cholesterol away from the arteries back to the liver where it is broken down. You can do a simple calculation to see if your level of cholesterol is dangerous. If you divide the total cholesterol by the HDL cholesterol and the result is less than 4.5, you are at lower risk to have a heart attack. The higher that number, the greater your risk.

You can do something to raise your HDL or "good" cholesterol. The best way is exercise. The more you do (within reason), the higher your HDL and the lower your risk of a heart attack.

High cholesterol is also a well-known effect of hypothyroidism. Moreover, high cholesterol is not only associated with coronary artery disease and heart attacks, but with peripheral vascular disease (leading to blocked blood flow to the arms and legs) and cerebral artery disease, which can lead to strokes.

The number of people with high cholesterol is far greater than the number of people who have hypothyroidism. Most abnormalities in cholesterol are due to excessive fat in the diet and lack of exercise

However, there may be many cases of undiagnosed hypothyroidism that do result in high cholesterol. Studies show that more than 10 percent of people with high cholesterol (levels over 200) have hypothyroidism. Most people with high cholesterol have never been tested for hypothyroidism, and most people do not know that hypothyroidism and high cholesterol have a connection in the first place.

When a patient with high cholesterol is diagnosed with hypothyroidism, the treatment is, of course, thyroid hormone. The results can be pretty dramatic with a major improvement in the fats in the blood. (This result may not be true for people with *subclinical hypothyroidism,* an elevated TSH level but a normal free T4.) Reduction in cholesterol by as much as 30 to 40 percent may follow the use of thyroid hormone in a person with hypothyroidism.

The explanation for the increase in cholesterol in hypothyroidism is that the metabolism (or breakdown) of cholesterol declines with hypothyroidism just as the metabolism of everything else in the body declines. However, the production of cholesterol remains the same, leading to a rise in the blood cholesterol.

If your cholesterol is elevated above 200, ask your doctor to check your thyroid function.

Moderating your sugar intake

The U.S. government guidelines recommend choosing beverages and foods to moderate your intake of sugars. There are many reasons for this recommendation:

- ✔ Sugary foods promote tooth decay.
- ✔ Sugary foods often contain few essential nutrients and replace those foods that have these nutrients.
- ✔ Sugary foods are the source of many calories. They are often eaten in an effort to avoid fatty foods, but you still end up with too many calories.

You can avoid these problems by keeping your portions of sugary foods like pies, cakes, candies, and cookies small. Substituting fruit for these sugary desserts will reduce sugar intake, provide a certain amount of sweetness for your sweet tooth, and provide other important nutrients all at once.

The biggest offender when it comes to eating lots of sugar with no nutrition is a bottle of soda. Unless it's diet soda, prepared with noncaloric sweeteners, the typical bottle of soda gives you a huge amount of sugar and nothing else. Even the flavored fruit sodas have this problem. Do yourself a favor and switch to water with lemon or lime or the diet sodas that have no sugar. Be sure to read the label to find out what you're drinking.

Choosing and preparing foods with less salt

The guideline regarding salt intake is meant to protect you from developing high blood pressure. The recommended amount of salt is a teaspoon, or 6 grams, daily. Most people eat twice as much as that, or more. One problem is that food manufacturers typically add a lot of salt to their foods. Avoid this by choosing low salt foods.

Another problem is that people are so used to picking up the salt shaker and heavily spraying their food with salt. The result is food that tastes like salt and not much else. Try your food without salt for a change. At first it may taste bland, but then you will begin to notice the subtle flavors of the food coming through. When you do, you may never want to go back to eating so much salt again.

Most recipes, especially in older cookbooks, recommend more salt than is necessary for proper preparation of the food. Try reducing the salt in the recipe by half. The food will probably cook just as well and the taste may even be superior. If you don't tell your family that you have reduced the salt, they'll probably never know.

In the United States and many other countries, iodized salt is the major source of iodine. That teaspoon of salt a day contains twice as much iodine as you are required to eat each day, so you could reduce your salt intake to a half teaspoon and still be assured of getting enough. If you eat one piece of bread, it contains just about your daily requirement of iodine. You do not need to eat excess salt to assure yourself of getting enough iodine.

Drinking alcohol in moderation

People who consume more than one or two drinks of alcohol a day or more than ten in a week should work to reduce those amounts. Like cigarettes, alcohol can damage your body in many ways. It raises your blood pressure, causes liver destruction, and promotes certain cancers. It provides no nutrition and often causes you to eat less of the foods you need for good nutrition. Severe alcoholism results in damage to the nervous system, vitamin deficiency diseases, anemia, and skin damage.

Alcohol also destroys families. When one or more members of a family are alcoholics, the incidence of divorce, accidents, suicide, loss of employment, and disease within that family is much greater than in families that do not have an alcoholic member. Alcoholism can also lead to impotency, making sexual relations impossible.

Keep in mind that alcohol in moderation can raise the level of HDL or "good" cholesterol in your body. Alcohol can also be a pleasant part of a meal and a key element in certain social scenes. Clearly, alcohol is not going to go away, but you must control its use.

Keeping foods safe to eat

To protect yourself from the chemicals that are sprayed on foods as they are grown and the chemicals present in the soil that fruits and vegetables are grown in, wash all fruits and vegetables before eating them. (Obviously, this does not eliminate chemicals inside the food.)

Proper refrigeration of foods that can spoil is essential. Raw meat, fish, and poultry must be kept in the refrigerator before cooking them thoroughly. Keep your hands clean when you handle these foods. And make sure that cutting boards and knives are cleaned well after you use them for cutting raw meats. The use of a mild bleach solution to cleanse cutting boards is also recommended.

After you cook food, if you want to save it for a later time, keep it in the refrigerator. Leaving it at room temperature allows bacteria to grow that may be present when the food is eaten again, even if it's reheated.

Making good food choices

You can easily choose to eat foods that contribute to better health and weight control over those that lead to illness and obesity. You just need to know how to substitute one for the other. In Table 19-2, I show you the wiser choices that you can make every day. By making these choices, you will notice little loss of taste but a definite improvement in your health and your ability to lose weight.

Table 19-2	Choosing Healthier Foods	
Food Group	*Better Choice*	*Worse Choice*
Breads	Whole-grain breads, whole-grain and bran cereals, rice, pasta	Refined-flour breads and cakes, croissants, cookies, pastries
Vegetables	Dark green, leafy vegetables; yellow-orange vegetables; cabbage; broccoli	Avocados, vegetables in butter or cream sauce
Fruits	Citrus fruits, berries, apples, pears	Coconut, fruit pies or pastries
Dairy	Low-fat cheese, low or non-fat milk, sherbet	Whole milk, butter, sweet cream, ice cream, cream cheese, hard cheeses
Meats	Lean meats, chicken, fresh fish, cooked dry beans and peas, egg whites	Fatty meats, lunch meats, tuna in oil, egg yolks (or whole eggs), sausages

Clarifying the Thyroid–Weight Connection

Certain misconceptions exist about how your thyroid reacts to weight loss, and how your weight reacts to a change in your thyroid function. In this section, I hope to dispel these misconceptions by showing you how your thyroid and your weight really interact.

Does my metabolism slow when I lose weight?

People who lose weight on a diet often regain the weight after a time. If you've had this experience, maybe you've heard that the reason you can't keep the weight off is that your thyroid and metabolism slow down after you've lost some pounds, so the weight comes back on more easily. This reasoning implies that your body establishes a "set point" weight and tries to maintain it by changing your thyroid function and your metabolism whenever you move away from that weight. The idea is that if you lose weight, your metabolic rate falls because your thyroid function declines. Researchers have studied this idea to determine its validity.

In a study in the *American Journal of Clinical Nutrition* in November 2000, researchers tested thyroid function and metabolic rates for 24 overweight women in the process of losing weight. When they were actively losing weight, the women's resting metabolic rates and free T3 hormone levels declined. But after they reached their normal weight, their free T3 levels and resting metabolic rate were normal as well. This study contradicts the idea of a "set point" weight.

If you are having trouble keeping off the weight you lose and your thyroid is functioning normally, this study shows that you can't blame your thyroid. You may want to take a closer look at your exercise and eating habits instead.

If I'm treated for hyperthyroidism, am I doomed to gain weight?

Many people who are treated for hyperthyroidism with radioactive iodine complain that they cannot lose weight after they become hypothyroid and are placed on thyroid hormone replacement. If this describes your situation, you should consider a number of possible explanations:

- You may not be taking enough thyroid hormones to replace your deficit. It is important to check that your thyroid-stimulating hormone (TSH) is in the normal range and ideally less than 2.5.

- You may need to take T3 hormone replacement as well as T4, even if your TSH is normal (see Chapter 4).

- You may be eating some food that interferes with thyroid hormone absorption, such as soy protein, around the time you take the thyroid hormone.

Then again, it's possible that none of the above can explain your weight gain. A study in the *Journal of the American College of Nutrition* in 1999 attempted to address this issue. The authors studied 10 people who were treated with radioactive iodine for hyperthyroidism. The researchers looked at the participants' total food energy intake; their T4, T3, and TSH levels; and their height and weight at the time of treatment and at 1, 2, 3, 6, and 12 months afterward. The participants' thyroid hormone levels declined in the first months of treatment but increased later. Even when thyroid hormone levels increased, the participants continued to gain weight. Interestingly, the average weight of the participants before the development of hyperthyroidism was about 170 pounds; at the time of treatment, 148 pounds; and after a year, about 168 pounds. Their final average weight was actually *lower* than their average weight before hyperthyroidism developed. The study concluded that weight gain after treatment of hyperthyroidism was initially due to a fall in the metabolic rate that accompanied the drop in thyroid hormone but later was due to food intake or lifestyle choices.

Another study in the *Journal of Clinical Endocrinology and Metabolism* in 1998 showed where the weight gain occurs in the body when hyperthyroidism is treated. The researchers showed that most of the weight gain in the first three months occurred as fat in the waist area and in muscle tissue, whereas weight gain later on was in the fat under the skin. This study shows very clearly that the weight loss that occurred before treatment for hyperthyroidism was loss of lean tissue, the muscle mass. (It is further proof that using excess thyroid hormone for weight loss leads to loss of muscle.)

Many people treated for hyperthyroidism gain more weight than they want to after treatment. In most cases, this occurs either because their thyroid hormone levels are not in the range they should be, or because they do not alter their eating and exercise habits after treatment. If you're in this situation, keep in mind that you probably increased your food intake and decreased your activity level when your body was hyperthyroid. You need to make lifestyle adjustments after treatment in order to bring your body back to its healthy weight.

The thyroid and celiac disease

Celiac disease is an autoimmune disease of the small intestine that results in poor absorption of fat, protein, carbohydrates, iron, and vitamins A, D, and K. The consequences of celiac disease are diarrhea, *osteomalacia* (poorly mineralized bone), signs of vitamin deficiency, and anemia. Studies have shown that as high as 21 percent of patients with celiac disease also have autoimmune hypothyroidism, and 3 percent of people with thyroid disease have celiac disease.

The treatment for celiac disease is to remove gluten from the patient's diet. Gluten is found in wheat, barley, oats, and rye, and as a filler in many prepared foods and medications. When gluten is removed from the diet, not only does the celiac disease disappear, but the patient's thyroid disease is cured as well.

A study in the *American Journal of Gastroenterology* in March 2001 found that out of 241 patients with celiac disease, 31 (13 percent) also had hypothyroidism. Of the 31, 29 had subclinical hypothyroidism with an elevation in TSH but a normal T4. When they were treated for a year by avoiding gluten in their diet and the celiac disease was cured, the thyroid abnormalities disappeared in all of them as well.

Thyroid disease is so commonly associated with celiac disease that everyone with celiac disease should be tested for thyroid disease. If present, both the celiac disease and the thyroid disorder may respond to gluten withdrawal.

Getting Enough Iodine in a Vegetarian Diet

Because iodine is a key element of thyroid hormones, iodine is a necessary part of your daily diet.

Vegetarians avoid eating the key foods that contain iodine, such as fish, seafood, eggs, meat, and milk. You must have sufficient iodine in your diet to have good thyroid health. A study of vegetarians in the *British Journal of Medicine* in December 1998 found that 63 percent of the females and 36 percent of the males had inadequate iodine intake.

If you follow a vegetarian diet, you may want to take iodized salt or iodine supplements. If you have any doubt about whether you're getting enough iodine, ask your doctor to check your iodine level (with a urine test). A teaspoon of salt a day or a piece or two of bread will take care of your iodine needs as a vegetarian.

Avoiding iodine before thyroid studies

The results of thyroid uptake studies are more valuable if the subjects avoid foods that contain iodine for a time before the test. The purpose of most such studies is to determine the size and shape of the thyroid and whether a given abnormality of the thyroid takes up iodine.

If you are being tested for hyperthyroidism, you don't have to avoid iodine. In fact, avoiding iodine may confuse the diagnosis because you are looking for abnormally high uptake of the iodine, and you do not want to artificially enhance the test results by following a low-iodine diet.

If you are having a thyroid scan done for reasons other than hyperthyroidism, follow a low-iodine diet for several days:

- ✔ Use only noniodized salt.
- ✔ Avoid milk or milk products.
- ✔ Avoid commercial vitamin preparations unless they definitely do not contain iodine.
- ✔ Steer clear of eggs.
- ✔ Don't eat seafood, fish, shellfish, seaweed, or kelp.
- ✔ Avoid cured or corned foods.
- ✔ Don't use bread products made with iodine dough conditioners.
- ✔ Avoid foods that contain Red Dye # 3, chocolate, molasses, or soy.

Exercising for Your Thyroid

If you're being successfully treated for a thyroid condition and tests show that you have normal thyroid function, you can exercise as much as you want. (Just be sure to listen to your body and slow down if you feel like you're overextending yourself.) You should be doing aerobic exercise, in which your heart is forced to beat faster, to keep your heart healthy and your body fat under control. You should also be doing strength training to retain and build muscle.

If you have a thyroid condition that hasn't yet been treated, you need to be aware of some special considerations regarding exercise. In this section, I discuss these situations and talk about how to use exercise to maximize your health in general.

Recognizing the natural consequences of aging

Don't confuse the natural effects of aging with the consequences of having thyroid disease. As you get older, your ability to do aerobic exercise is going to decrease, as is your strength. If you go to the gym for the first time in years and find that you can't last as long on the treadmill as you used to, chances are that your thyroid isn't the culprit.

Your ability to take in oxygen is a measure of your physical condition. Your oxygen uptake peaks around age 25, and after that, it steadily declines no matter what you do to prevent it. Your strength also seems to peak around the same time, but it remains more or less the same until around age 40, when it starts to decline steadily. We all lose about 25 percent of our maximum strength by age 65. We also lose flexibility with aging — our tendons, ligaments, and joint capsules become stiffer.

You have certainly heard the old saying, "You will only be young once." Take my word for it: It's true.

At any age, you can maximize your strength, your stamina, and your flexibility by doing plenty of exercise. By plenty, I mean at least 30 minutes, 4 or more times per week.

Working out with hypothyroidism

When you have an underactive thyroid, your ability to exercise is limited by the fatigue that accompanies this condition. After you have begun taking the proper replacement dose of thyroid hormone, you should be able to exercise normally. But if you still can't exercise because of fatigue, consider the two common reasons:

✔ You may not be receiving sufficient thyroid hormone so your TSH is between 0.5 and 2.5. If your symptoms linger even after taking the hormone replacement, don't settle for a TSH of 3 or higher.

✔ You may need to take T3 hormone in addition to T4 to fully replace your missing thyroid function.

Hypothyroidism does affect the functioning of your heart, which can become apparent during exercise. If you're being treated with thyroid hormone, your heart function should return to normal (assuming that you don't have any other heart conditions).

Heart function during exercise may actually be a greater issue for patients with *subclinical hypothyroidism* (where your TSH is elevated but your free T4 is normal), because these patients are not necessarily treated with thyroid hormone. (See Chapter 15 for a detailed discussion of the debate over treatment.) Subclinical hypothyroidism is associated with mild abnormalities in the heart, which are not measurable when you are resting but are detected when you exercise. The normal heart's adaptation to effort is diminished in subclinical hypothyroidism. Subclinical hypothyroidism also results in a rise in the form of cholesterol that leads to heart attacks and a fall in the form that is protective against heart attacks. Some thyroid specialists believe that these subtle changes are reason enough to treat subclinical hypothyroidism with thyroid hormone.

The muscles of a person with subclinical hypothyroidism show abnormal energy metabolism that leads to early fatigue, which is also corrected by thyroid hormone. The ability of blood vessels to open up to allow more blood flow is also impaired. This is further evidence of the need for treatment, particularly before the condition worsens.

Exercising with hyperthyroidism

If you are hyperthyroid, your heart rate and the amount of blood pumped per heartbeat are both elevated when you are resting, but they do not respond to exercise in a normal fashion. After normal thyroid function is achieved through treatment, these abnormalities disappear.

Careful study of the hearts of hyperthyroid patients shows that their resting heart rates are abnormally high, as are the frequent occurrences of abnormal heart rhythms. The size of the heart is increased as a result of abnormal thickening of the heart muscle.

With exercise, the hyperthyroid heart cannot increase its workload the way that a normal heart can. The result is that the hyperthyroid person cannot exercise as long as she used to, and her peak level of exercise is reduced. This is true even in subclinical hyperthyroidism, where the TSH is suppressed below the normal range but the free T4 remains normal. When the beta blocker propranolol is given to slow the heart, the patient feels an improvement in exercise capacity.

An elderly person with hyperthyroidism must be especially careful with exercise because she has an increased risk of heart failure and she may experience abnormal heart rhythms (which may not improve even when the hyperthyroidism is brought under control). Chest pain can get worse as hyperthyroidism continues.

Not only heart muscle but also skeletal (arm, leg, and trunk) muscles are abnormal in hyperthyroidism. Hyperthyroid skeletal muscle requires more energy to perform the same amount of work as healthy muscle. As a result, it can be fatigued much earlier.

Meeting your minimal exercise needs

While you are recovering from hypothyroidism or hyperthyroidism, you may not be able to do much exercise and certainly not the amount necessary for good health. After you are cured, however, you want to get up to speed.

You want to do two types of exercise:

- ✔ **Aerobic exercise:** To improve heart and lung function and raise the healthy cholesterol
- ✔ **Anaerobic exercise:** To strengthen muscles and increase stamina

Any exercise that gets the heart beating faster for a sustained period is aerobic exercise. Doctors used to recommend a formula for determining the ideal heart rate during exercise: Subtract your age from 220, and your ideal heart rate is 60 to 75 percent of that number. Now we know that many people can sustain aerobic exercise at higher heart rates. Perhaps the best way to know whether you're meeting your exercise goals is to rank the exercise as follows: very, very light; very light; fairly light; somewhat hard; very hard; and very, very hard. If you stay at the level of *somewhat hard* while you get into shape, you'll be doing the right amount of aerobic exercise.

Aerobic exercise should be sustained for 20 to 30 minutes every day. By doing this, despite the normal loss of exercise capacity with aging, you are maximizing what you have and adding significant time to your life.

Don't forget to do muscle strengthening exercises as well. Using light weights of ten to fifteen pounds, three times a week, you want to do three or four different exercises to work your arms and legs and strengthen your back.

For a complete program of exercise instruction, see my previous book, *Diabetes For Dummies,* as well as *Weight Training For Dummies* (both published by Hungry Minds, Inc.).

Leptin: The New Hormone on the Block

Leptin is a relatively new hormone that has an important role in normal thyroid function. First described in 1994, *leptin* is a hormone made by fat cells that is a major regulator of body weight. As your body fat goes up, the leptin in your body increases.

When a person fasts, he or she has a fall in T3 and TSH. A fall in leptin may be responsible for this, which could explain a decline in weight loss that occurs over time in a fasting individual. In the future, the use of leptin during a diet may promote increased weight loss.

This section explains the brief history of our knowledge of leptin and what we know so far about its relationship with thyroid hormone.

Learning the functions of leptin

The first studies of this hormone were conducted on a strain of obese rats, which were found to have a genetic mutation that resulted in failure of leptin production. Administering leptin to these mice resulted in weight loss — the mice reduced their food intake and had increased energy. The same thing was found when leptin was given to normal-weight mice — they lost fat mass. Leptin was then discovered in human beings and was hailed as the obesity gene. Unfortunately, injections of leptin in human beings did not lead to substantial weight loss.

Obesity is not the result of a genetic mutation in the leptin gene. However, several families have been found to have a mutation of the leptin gene that leads to severe obesity at a young age. This gene is a *recessive trait,* meaning that family members who have only one abnormal leptin gene instead of two do not show the disease. When people with the disease are given leptin, they experience significant weight loss and the reversal of metabolic abnormalities.

Further studies showed that leptin was doing more than just signaling the body that it had too much fat. When researchers compared body-fat percentages and leptin levels of women and men, women were found to have leptin levels that were as much as two to three times that of men. But even though women typically have more fat mass than men, this result does not fully explain the difference. Studies have now shown that the female sex hormone, estrogen, stimulates leptin production, while the male sex hormone, testosterone, suppresses leptin.

Researchers have known that girls go into puberty when they reach a certain weight. Puberty begins when a hormone from the *hypothalamus,* a part of the brain, begins to be released. This hormone is called *gonadotrophin-releasing hormone* (GnRH). The question arose, what was the signal to release GnRH? The presence of leptin proved to be the answer to that question because it clearly indicates when the fat mass is sufficient for puberty to begin.

Interacting with thyroid hormone

Leptin has now been shown to interact with several other hormones in the body, especially insulin, which appears to have an important place in regulating leptin secretion. Leptin interacts with the adrenal gland and growth hormone as well. Because thyroid hormone increases the metabolic rate, which increases the body temperature, researchers thought that leptin (which also regulates metabolism and body temperature) might interact with thyroid hormone.

It has now been shown that leptin helps to regulate the part of the brain that releases *thyrotrophin-releasing hormone* (TRH), and it also regulates the release of thyroid-stimulating hormone. When a person fasts, both the thyroid hormone and leptin concentrations fall. If leptin is given to the fasting individual, the TSH and the T4 hormone return to normal.

On the other hand, thyroid hormone has been found to control leptin production to some extent. In animals without thyroids, leptin is increased, but when thyroid hormone is replaced, leptin is suppressed. So far in humans, thyroid hormone has not been shown to cause either a rise or a fall in leptin concentration.

Our understanding of the role of leptin is at an early stage. Much more will be learned in the next few years. Leptin's place in thyroid disease is just starting to be clarified; stay tuned.

Part V
The Part of Tens

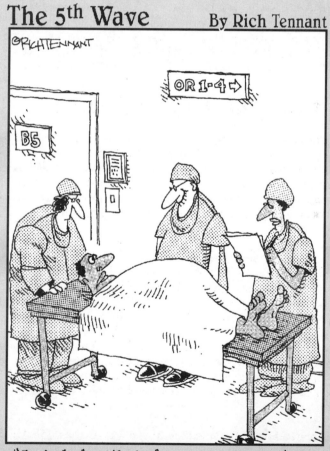

"Included with today's surgery, we're offering a manicure, pedicure, haircut, and ear wax flush for just $49.95."

In this part . . .

As you would expect, a part of your body as important as the thyroid prompts all sorts of myths and mistaken ideas. Here you find the ones I consider the most important (and possibly the most damaging if you believe them). The final chapter shows you what you can do to make sure that you maximize your thyroid health in ten easy steps.

Chapter 20

Ten Myths about Thyroid Health

Thanks to the Internet, you have access to incredible amounts of information about your thyroid. Unfortunately, much (perhaps most) of it is not accurate. Much of what you read online is based on the experiences and opinions of one or a few people who took this or that medicine or herb and got better in two weeks. It's important to maintain a healthy degree of skepticism.

In this chapter, I try to clear up some commonly held myths concerning the thyroid and its diseases.

I'm Hypothyroid, So I Can't Lose Weight

If you have hypothyroidism, or if you've been treated for a thyroid condition and the cure resulted in your becoming hypothyroid, you may find that you have a hard time losing weight. The myth is that you can't lose weight if you have hypothyroidism, even when it's properly treated.

The truth is that a large percentage of people who are being successfully treated for hypothyroidism weigh almost the same after being treated as they did before they developed the disease.

I have occasionally seen hypothyroid patients — mostly elderly people — who actually lose weight, rather than gain it, after they receive replacement thyroid hormone. This occurs when a patient is receiving poor nutrition, which is made worse by the complacency that can accompany hypothyroidism, because he or she may not take in enough calories.

Keep in mind that hypothyroidism is associated with fatigue. Many patients with hypothyroidism reduce their physical activity as a result. They may not restore their previous level of activity after the hypothyroidism is treated properly.

If you struggle to lose the weight that you've gained after becoming hypothyroid, and if your activity level has remained the same, it's possible that your thyroid treatment is inadequate (which can be determined with a TSH test) or that you need to take T3 replacement hormone in addition to T4 (see Chapter 5).

There's also the possibility that another autoimmune condition is present. Because the most common cause of hypothyroidism is autoimmune thyroiditis (see Chapter 5), your doctor should look for diabetes mellitus type 1 or autoimmune adrenal insufficiency (Addison's disease — failure to make the hormone cortisol), among other conditions. This is easily done by a blood glucose test for diabetes or a serum cortisol level for autoimmune adrenal insufficiency.

Your thyroid health and the Internet

You are not completely on your own when it comes to reading thyroid sites on the Net. If you are lucky enough to find a statement on a Web site indicating that it adheres to the Health on the Net Foundation Code of Conduct (HONcode), you can feel sure that the information is accurate. In addition, at the back of this book in Appendix B, and on my Web site (www.drrubin.com), I have listed sites that I consider authoritative and accurate. Just go to my site, click on Useful Addresses on the home page, select Thyroid Sites on the next page, and read to your heart's content.

The Health on the Net Foundation has established a set of principles that any site on the Internet can adhere to. A site that follows the HONcode principles has agreed to the following:

Principle 1: Medical advice will be given by qualified professionals (or the site will state that this is not the case).

Principle 2: The information supports, but does not replace, the patient/physician relationship.

Principle 3: Confidentiality of visitors to the site is respected.

Principle 4: Information is supported by references.

Principle 5: Claims about the benefits of specific treatments are supported by references.

Principle 6: Information is provided in the clearest possible manner, with contacts provided for more information — including the Webmaster's e-mail address.

Principle 7: Support for the site is clearly identified (especially commercial support).

Principle 8: If a site is supported by advertising, it's clearly stated, along with the advertising policy. Advertising is clearly differentiated from nonadvertising material.

Conducting proper medical studies

The myths in this chapter have been found not to be true by scientists who conducted studies using control groups (people who did not get active medicine or treatment but thought they did) and treatment groups (people who got the active medicine or treatment but weren't certain that they did). In studies like this, even the doctors administering the treatment or medicine do not know who is getting real treatment and who is not. Only by conducting studies this way is there a fair comparison between groups. This is the famous *double blind placebo controlled study,* and it's arranged in the following manner:

✔ No patient knows what he or she is getting, nor does the doctor, but all get something — either real treatment or a placebo.

✔ The benefits for the patient getting the real treatment must be significantly better than those for the patient getting a placebo.

✔ The side effects for each group should be about equal so the patient with the disease is not having many more side effects than the person serving as a control.

The bottom line is that we all follow the principle of conservation of energy. If we take in too much energy compared to what we need, we gain weight. If we take in too little energy compared to what we need, we lose weight.

Another truth is that our metabolic rate declines, as does our tendency to move around, as we age. Both changes tend to make weight loss more difficult, but it's still possible.

If you have had hypothyroidism and are on the proper dose of thyroid hormone, you will be able to lose weight with sufficient diet and exercise.

I'm Hyperthyroid, So I Can't Gain Weight

The myth that hyperthyroidism is always accompanied by weight loss is a source of confusion in making an accurate diagnosis. Although the majority of patients do lose weight when they become hyperthyroid, some patients actually gain weight — the elderly, in particular.

A study published in the *Journal of the American Geriatric Society* in 1996 compared 19 classical signs of hyperthyroidism in older patients and younger patients. Three signs were found in more than 50 percent of older patients: rapid heartbeat, fatigue, and weight loss. However, some people experienced no weight loss or weight gain. Seven signs were found less frequently in older patients than in younger, while only two signs — loss of appetite and an irregular heart rhythm — were found more often in the older patients. Overall, of the 19 classical clinical signs, older people had only 6 of them on average, while younger people had 11.

Another study published in *Thyroidology* in 1992 showed very similar results. It also emphasized the importance of checking levels of thyroid hormones and TSH in the elderly population before making a diagnosis of hyperthyroidism.

Weight loss, as well as other symptoms of hyperthyroidism, may not always be present, especially in the elderly population. The best solution is to get thyroid blood tests every 5 years, beginning at age 35.

Breastfeeding and Antithyroid Pills Don't Mix

For years, doctors advised women who were treated with antithyroid pills for hyperthyroidism during pregnancy not to breastfeed. The fear was that the medication would enter the baby's circulation through the breast milk and make the baby hypothyroid. This has now been found to be a myth.

Two important studies have shown that this belief was incorrect. In one study published in the *Journal of Clinical Endocrinology and Metabolism,* 88 mothers were given one of the two major antithyroid drugs, methimazole, for 12 months. The levels of methimazole in the babies' blood were measured. In addition, the babies were tested for thyroid function, urinary iodine, thyroid autoantibodies, intelligence quotient (IQ), and verbal and functional ability. All of the babies of treated mothers had normal thyroid function. They grew normally, and their IQ, verbal, and functional tests were identical to children who breast-fed from mothers without hyperthyroidism.

In a second study, the other major antithyroid drug, propylthiouricil (PTU), was given to breastfeeding mothers; some took as much as 750 milligrams of PTU daily. Again the thyroid function tests of the babies were entirely normal, as was the babies' development.

A hyperthyroid mother taking methimazole or propylthiouricil to control her hyperthyroidism may safely breastfeed her new baby.

Brand Name Thyroid Hormone Pills Are Best

Because the number of people taking thyroid replacement hormone in the United States and throughout the world is enormous, the amount of money spent on thyroid hormone replacement pills is also huge. The company that captures the largest share of the market is going to make its stockholders very happy.

The myth is that generic preparations of thyroxine (T4 hormone) are not equal in potency to brand name thyroxine, are not standardized over time, and should not be used in the treatment of hypothyroidism.

This myth began, as so many do, with research that was correct at the time but is now outdated. In 1980, an article appeared in the *Journal of the American Medical Association* showing that generic preparations were not equal to brand name thyroxine. Sometimes the generic preparations were weaker and sometimes they were stronger; they were not uniform from lot to lot. This type of information continued to appear in medical literature as late as 1995.

However, a study that was completed in 1990 — but did not appear until 1997 in the *Journal of the American Medical Association* — looked at the problem again. Twenty women who were being successfully treated for hypothyroidism were put on four different preparations at the same dosage for six weeks at a time. Blood tests taken during this study showed that there was absolutely no difference in any of the preparations. All the preparations met the Food and Drug Administration criterion for equivalent activity. The conclusion was that the preparations, including two brand names and two generics, were sufficiently equal in their activity and there was no reason to choose any one over the others. This study, I am happy to add, was performed by my great thyroid mentor, Dr. Francis Greenspan, among others.

It has been alleged that the last study was originally paid for by one of the brand name companies making thyroid hormone replacement, and when the study did not show that theirs was a better product, they suppressed its results.

Generic thyroid preparations save you money and can be used interchangeably with brand name thyroxine. Because hypothyroidism may not be a stable condition, you still want to have your thyroid function checked regularly (perhaps yearly).

1 Have to Take Thyroid Medication for Life

Many patients are told that once they are on thyroid hormone replacement, they'll be taking it for life. For many people, this is true. Any treatment that removes or destroys much of the thyroid (such as surgery or radioactive iodine) will require treatment with thyroxine (T4 hormone) for life. However, in certain situations, hypothyroidism is temporary; you may need thyroxine for a time, but you will later stop taking it. Sometimes it may be obvious that you no longer need the medication, but other times you and your doctor may need to attempt a trial period off thyroid for 4 to 6 weeks to see if you still need it.

The following are some of the conditions that require thyroid hormone replacement for a limited amount of time. Each is explained in detail in Chapter 11:

- ✔ *Subacute thyroiditis* causes the temporary breakdown of thyroid cells and the release of thyroxine from the thyroid. As this condition improves, thyroxine begins to be made and stored again, and oral thyroxine is no longer necessary.

- ✔ *Silent* and *postpartum thyroiditis* also cause temporary loss of thyroxine, which is restored with time.

- ✔ *Acute thyroiditis* occasionally requires temporary treatment with thyroid hormone.

The major diagnosis that means you may or may not be taking thyroid hormone pills for life is chronic thyroiditis (see Chapter 5). This condition is the result of antibodies that block TSH from sufficiently stimulating the thyroid to produce enough thyroid hormone. Occasionally, levels of blocking antibodies fall. The only way you will know if this happens is by measuring the antibodies (which is not well standardized) or stopping the thyroid hormone and testing thyroid function 4 to 6 weeks later. If your thyroid function remains normal, you may not have to take thyroxine any longer.

Depending on your diagnosis, you may be able to stop thyroid hormone treatment at some point. It's well worth checking, particularly if you are young (under 40).

Natural Thyroid Hormones Are Better Than Synthetic Hormones

The first thyroid hormones used to treat people with low thyroid function were extracted from the thyroids of animals and called *desiccated thyroid* (see Chapter 5). After decades of use, desiccated thyroid was replaced by synthetic thyroid hormones made in the laboratory. Some holdouts still believe that desiccated thyroid is superior to synthetic thyroxine (T4 hormone) for treating hypothyroidism.

As long ago as 1978, an article in the *American Journal of Medicine* was titled "Why does anyone still use desiccated thyroid USP?" The article declared desiccated thyroid an obsolete therapy. The hormone extracted from animals has plenty of problems:

- ✔ Desiccated thyroid cannot be standardized from dose to dose because one animal has a different amount of the thyroid hormones in its thyroid than the next animal.

- ✔ Desiccated thyroid has impurities that may cause immune reactions.

- ✔ The use of desiccated thyroid confuses the thyroid testing. If only the total T4 hormone is measured, that result will often be low because of the large amount of T3 in the medication. The patient may receive even more thyroid hormone and actually become hyperthyroid.

- ✔ Not only does the dose of T4 and T3 supplied by desiccated thyroid vary from pill to pill, but it also does not provide the same levels as what the normal thyroid releases.

These problems have had their consequences in the past. Patients have been undertreated or overtreated by different preparations of desiccated thyroid. Some patients have been found to be hyperthyroid for a few hours a day due to the large amount of T3 in some desiccated thyroid pills.

One thing to be said for desiccated thyroid is that it does contain some T3, which most synthetic hormone replacements don't have. However, a synthetic preparation of T3 does exist, and it's far superior to the mixture in desiccated thyroid.

Synthetic thyroxine is currently the medication of choice in the treatment of hypothyroidism. In the future, a combination of T4 and T3 in the exact ratio that it leaves the thyroid will replace T4 alone.

Thyroid Disease Is Catching

It's not hard to understand why this myth became so entrenched in the minds of the public. Most thyroid disease is inherited; so the likelihood of finding the same disease in two sisters or a mother and her daughter is relatively high, suggesting that their physical closeness to one another causes them to have the same disease. Furthermore, in areas where people don't consume enough iodine, practically everyone has thyroid disease — again suggesting that it may be catching.

Another situation that seems to suggest that thyroid disease is catching is the occurrence of thyroid disease after large-scale radiation exposure. Just about everyone comes down with some illness in that situation. Children, especially, often develop goiters, nodules, and thyroid cancers.

An understanding of the way these diseases develop quickly clarifies the situation:

- ✔ The hereditary thyroid diseases affect the females of a family, usually sparing the males.

- ✔ After iodine is supplied, the incidence of thyroid disease rapidly declines in iodine-deficient areas.

- ✔ Children who take iodine pills or avoid exposure to radioactive iodine generally will not get thyroid diseases, while those who do not, will.

You cannot catch thyroid disease, nor can you give it to someone else in the way that germs are passed from person to person.

Iodine Deficiency Is a Medical Problem

Because iodine deficiency (see Chapter 12) causes hypothyroidism, goiter, and cretinism (when severe), you would think that it's a clear-cut disease that should respond to medical treatment with iodine. If this were so, the disease would have disappeared years ago.

As with any major medical problem (like AIDS, breast cancer, and prostate cancer), iodine deficiency is a social, economic, and political problem as much as, or more than, it is a medical problem.

To begin with, an understanding about the cause of hypothyroidism in iodine-deficient areas is often lacking. The people are poor, work very hard, and have little time for the intricacies of the cause of disease. Their poverty means that they cannot afford to pay for nurses to give them medication or inject them with iodized oil. They do not understand that certain foods, like cassava, worsen the problem, so they continue to consume large quantities of them.

Often the local or federal government pumps in lots of money to improve the situation by providing iodine supplementation. But it provides no punishment for those who do not follow the regulations. Manufacturers may fail to put any iodine into their so-called "iodized" salt and claim the subsidies for it anyway. Much of that money disappears after it leaves government control.

Sometimes attempts to solve the problem run up against the realities of salt production. This has been the case in Indonesia, for example, where salt is made by numerous salt farmers rather than a centralized salt production facility (as is done in China). It was easier and more productive to alter the salt production to make enough iodized salt in China than it was in Indonesia.

When there's a tremendous need for a substance like iodine, the cheats try to profit from people's misery. They charge more for iodized salt and then fail to actually iodize the salt. They also underprice the government's iodized salt so that people buy their salt rather than true iodized salt from the government.

The instability of poor governments also plays a role. When the problem of iodine deficiency was recognized in Communist East Germany, iodine was provided and the disease was brought under fairly good control. After the reunification of East and West Germany, the combined government neglected the problem, and iodine deficiency began to reappear.

The solution to a clearly medical problem like iodine deficiency may have to involve social, cultural, and economic changes that populations often resist, making a cure exceedingly difficult.

The Higher My Autoantibody Levels, the Worse My Thyroid Disease

This myth derives from a phenomenon that seems obvious: The more you have of something that denotes a disease, the worse that disease must be. For example, if your temperature is 102 degrees Fahrenheit, you are probably sicker than someone whose temperature is only 99 degrees Fahrenheit. When it comes to thyroid autoantibodies, this does not seem to be the case.

When levels of autoantibodies are measured and compared with the severity of a patient's thyroid disease, there is no correlation. Some of the sickest patients with hyperthyroidism due to Graves' disease have relatively low levels of autoantibodies, while people with milder cases of Graves' may have high levels.

Adding to the confusion is the fact that the disappearance of thyroid autoantibodies after treatment with antithyroid drugs is a marker for improvement and suggests that the disease will not recur.

It's also true that very low levels of autoantibodies are often found in elderly women. But unless those women have abnormal thyroid function tests, the autoantibodies have little importance. Although people with low levels of autoantibodies should be retested occasionally, they don't require treatment unless a thyroid condition develops.

Autoantibody levels should not be compared between laboratories. There is little consistency in the methods by which the tests are done, so a level of a thousand at one laboratory means something very different from a level of a thousand at another laboratory.

Very high thyroid autoantibody levels do not indicate that you have a bad case of autoimmune thyroiditis. They simply confirm the diagnosis if other signs and symptoms exist.

Clinical Symptoms Are More Reliable Than Blood Tests

Thyroid disease can be very confusing. In certain age groups, particularly the elderly, the expected signs and symptoms may not exist. Sometimes, opposite symptoms are found. For example, some people gain weight as a result of hyperthyroidism.

Many people, including some physicians, believe that clinical signs and symptoms are more accurate than laboratory tests when diagnosing thyroid conditions.

What would someone who relies on symptoms do with an elderly woman who is apathetic, does not have an enlarged thyroid, and is depressed, but has a free T4 level of 3.5 and a TSH of less than 0.3? Her clinical signs and symptoms point to hypothyroidism, but her tests show hyperthyroidism. Relying on symptoms alone, a doctor might give this patient thyroid hormone replacement. Lots of luck.

I have relied upon thyroid function tests to diagnose disorders of thyroid function for 27 years. Especially in the last decade, as the TSH test has become more accurate and the free T4 and free T3 have become available, I have felt extremely confident that I have the right diagnosis.

The proof of the pudding is in the eating. When I treat patients with confusing clinical signs according to their lab test results rather than their clinical findings, they invariably get better.

One of the problems is that signs and symptoms of hypothyroidism can be very subtle, just like many other diseases. The signs and symptoms mimic those of diseases like depression, menopause, and aging.

Another problem is the placebo effect of any drug. If you give a group of patients a drug that's not supposed to have any effect on the disease in question, a few of them will get better. This does not mean that the drug is the reason they improved.

A good physician bases his or her treatment on evidence-based medicine. This means that single instances of improvement do not prove that a treatment is correct; they could just as easily mean that the original diagnosis was wrong.

Do not allow yourself to be treated by a doctor for a thyroid disease, such as hyperthyroidism or hypothyroidism, unless the thyroid function tests confirm the diagnosis.

Chapter 21

Ten Ways to Maximize Thyroid Health

*W*e have come a long way together. Now it's time to put the icing on the cake, or perhaps the exclamation point at the end of the sentence. In this chapter, I discuss the steps you can take to ensure your best thyroid function. You may have thought that there was little you could do — that your thyroid, like the Mississippi River, would just keep rolling along. As I show you here, you can do a lot to maximize thyroid health.

The things you can do fall into several categories. You can make sure that thyroid testing is done at the right intervals. You can do some self-examination to determine whether the shape of your thyroid is normal. You can make sure that you are getting the proper nutrients so that your thyroid can make its hormones in sufficient quantities. And perhaps most important of all, you can be knowledgeable about all the new discoveries concerning thyroid health and disease that appear on an almost daily basis.

By doing these things, you are doing all that you can to take care of that little gland that weighs less than an ounce but plays such an important role in your life and your health.

Screening at Appropriate Intervals

Many symptoms of hypothyroidism are subtle or are similar to symptoms of aging or menopause (see Chapter 5). Hyperthyroidism can also be tricky because symptoms may not be prominent (especially in elderly people), and sometimes symptoms appear to point toward an underactive thyroid even though the thyroid is overactive (see Chapter 18).

The most common form of thyroid disease is autoimmune thyroiditis. It probably affects 10 percent of the population of the United States, although only a small fraction of people with this disease actually develop hypothyroidism.

Hypothyroidism often begins when a woman is in her 30s. For this reason, and because of the confusion that can exist between the diagnosis and the signs and symptoms a patient experiences, doctors recommend that you start screening for abnormal thyroid function at age 35 and continue at 5-year intervals for the rest of your life. Of course, if tests reveal a thyroid condition, testing will be done much more frequently.

Screening is done by a blood test, the TSH (thyroid-stimulating hormone) test. Although the normal range is usually given as 0.5 to 5, the true normal range may be narrower, 0.5 to 2.5 (see Chapter 5). If your doctor tells you that your screening test was normal but you still have symptoms consistent with hypothyroidism, ask the doctor for the exact number of your TSH. If it's above 2.5, ask your doctor to consider giving you a trial of treatment with thyroid hormone replacement.

Checking Thyroid Function As Your Body Changes

If you are taking thyroid hormone treatment, you are on a fixed dose of medication. However, many physical states, particularly pregnancy (see Chapter 16), create chemical changes in your body that can alter the amount of thyroid hormone that you need to maintain normal function. The same is true as you get older.

Chemical changes that cause you to make more thyroid-binding proteins (see Chapter 4) require you to take an increased dose of thyroid medication. Any condition that increases your estrogens is an example, such as pregnancy and taking oral contraceptive pills. As more thyroid-binding proteins are made, more of your dose of thyroid is bound to the proteins and less is available to enter your cells. You must increase your dose of thyroid hormone. Blood tests determine when you again have enough.

Chemical changes that cause you to make less thyroid-binding proteins will require a decreased dose of thyroid hormone. If you take androgens (see Chapter 10) or have a disease that causes androgens to be produced excessively, you may need your dosage of thyroid hormone reduced. Less thyroid-binding protein means less binding of your thyroid dose, so more is available to enter cells. If you don't reduce your dose of thyroid hormone in this circumstance, you could become hyperthyroid.

Another situation that occurs in pregnancy is the reduction in autoimmunity (see Chapter 16). If you are being treated for hyperthyroidism with antithyroid pills, you may need a lower dose or none at all until the pregnancy is completed. Then you will need treatment again.

During times of major body change such as pregnancy or illness, your need for thyroid hormone or antithyroid medication may change. The only way to be sure you are on the right dose is to have thyroid function tests at regular intervals, usually every three months.

Performing a "Neck Check"

The American Association of Clinical Endocrinologists (AACE), recognizing that many people have thyroid disease that's not diagnosed, has proposed that everyone take the thyroid "Neck Check." Details may be found at their Web site, www.aace.com.

AACE urges everyone to "think thyroid." Its campaign for thyroid month in 2001 (thyroid month is January of each year) was to "think thyroid at critical life stages." This refers to the times of life that are covered in this book in Chapters 16 through 18.

Five steps are involved in doing a Neck Check. You need a hand-held mirror and a glass of water. The steps are:

1. Hold the mirror in your hand, focusing on the area of your neck just below the Adam's apple and immediately above the collarbone. Your thyroid is located in this area of your neck.

2. While focusing on this area in the mirror, tip your head back.

3. Take a drink of water and swallow.

4. As you swallow, look at your neck. Check for any bulges or protrusions in this area when you swallow. *Reminder:* Don't confuse the Adam's apple with the thyroid gland. The thyroid gland is located farther down on your neck, closer to the collarbone. You may want to repeat this process several times.

5. If you do see any bulges or protrusions in this area, see your physician. You may have an enlarged thyroid gland or a thyroid nodule and should be checked to determine whether cancer is present or if treatment for thyroid disease is needed.

You can detect abnormalities in the size and shape of your thyroid gland. If you think you have an enlarged thyroid, seek your doctor's help to determine whether there's any problem.

Getting Enough Iodine to Satisfy Your Thyroid

Iodine deficiency in the United States was once thought to be a thing of the past. With iodized salt and the addition of iodine to bread, there were no recognized cases of hypothyroidism due to lack of iodine in the U.S. for some time. In the 1970s and 1980s, in fact, doctors were concerned more about the overuse of iodine than the underuse. A study by the Michigan State Department of Health provided dramatic evidence of the benefit of the iodization of salt. The study indicated that in 1924, 39 percent of all children in several counties in Michigan were found to have a *goiter,* an enlarged thyroid. After salt was iodized, the numbers dropped to 10 percent by 1928 and 0.5 percent by 1951.

But a study in the *Journal of Clinical Endocrinology and Metabolism* in October, 1998 showed that the urinary excretion of iodine, a well-established method for monitoring sufficient iodine intake (see Chapter 12), had fallen by half compared to earlier times in the United States. Twelve percent of Americans had low iodine concentration in their urine compared to 1974, when the percentage was less than 1. Europe has also seen an increase in cases of iodine deficiency that has resulted in adding more iodine to table salt and monitoring more carefully the population's iodine intake. The major reasons for the decline seem to be a reduction in the addition of iodine to salt as well as a reduction of amounts of iodine in bread.

If you are a vegetarian, you may not eat the foods that are the major sources of iodine in the diet, namely fish and, to a lesser extent, meat, eggs, and milk. There's little iodine in fruits and vegetables.

Because our population is very concerned about high blood pressure, your doctor may urge you not to add salt to your food, because salt raises the blood pressure. However, the American Heart Association's nutritional recommendations are to limit salt intake to less than 6 grams daily, slightly more than a teaspoon. This amount contains plenty of iodine for your diet.

How do you act when you receive contradictory recommendations from health professionals? ("You need sufficient iodine." "Don't eat salt!") You can certainly use a small quantity of salt daily, and this contains enough iodine for your needs because 1 teaspoon of salt contains about 400 micrograms of iodine. Or you can eat a couple slices of bread each day. Each slice of bread contains about 150 micrograms of iodine. The recommended intake of iodine daily is 150 to 200 micrograms.

Stopping Thyroid Medication, If Possible

During my many years of medical practice, I have seen numerous people who were taking thyroid hormone who had never been tested with thyroid function tests. They had developed symptoms of fatigue or had gained a few pounds and had been put on medication. Most of these patients, when taken off thyroid hormone, proved to have normal thyroid function on their own. Often, if they were questioned as to whether the thyroid hormone had made a difference, they admitted that they were still fatigued and still had trouble losing weight, even on the medication. These people should never have been placed on thyroid hormone in the first place, but should certainly have had a trial off of thyroid hormone replacement over the years.

You are always better off if you let your normal body thyroid physiology work for you than if you try to replace it with an external source of thyroid hormones.

Another group of patients, who have been put on thyroid hormone replacement because of laboratory evidence of low thyroid function, may also get off thyroid hormone at some point. These are patients who have hypothyroidism due to chronic thyroiditis (see Chapter 5). Their hypothyroidism is the result of antibodies that block the action of thyroid-stimulating hormone. Up to 25 percent of these patients may be able to come off treatment. It's possible over time that the level of these blocking antibodies could fall to the point that the thyroid gland is able to make its own thyroid hormone. It's certainly worthwhile to try to stop the thyroid hormone after a few years of treatment to see if the thyroid can function on its own.

If you have hypothyroidism due to chronic thyroiditis and have been taking thyroid hormone pills for a few years, ask your doctor if you can stop the thyroid hormone replacement for a month and check your thyroid function tests.

Using Both Types of Thyroid Hormone

The thyroid gland makes two different thyroid hormones, T4, the major component, and T3, considered to be the active form of thyroid hormone but made in much lower amounts by the gland (see Chapter 3).

Because drug manufacturers have had the ability to synthesize it, T4 is the only treatment given when patients need thyroid hormone. It's given so that a patient's TSH level returns to normal, as does the free T4 in the blood. This means that most people who are treated for hypothyroidism have a deficiency of T3.

In practical terms, over the years this has not proven to be a significant problem. However, I have noted in my thyroid practice, as have other specialists, that a few patients continue to complain of symptoms of low thyroid function despite normal laboratory test results. These patients may improve if T3 is added to their treatment.

It's difficult to measure this kind of improvement objectively because the test results remain in the normal range. This is a case where I have been willing to accept the subjective symptoms of the patient indicating that he or she feels better on the combination therapy compared to T4 alone.

This is still a gray area in medicine. I have seen a handful of patients who did not feel better regardless of how much T3 was added, even though their thyroid tests were normal.

I hope that in the future we will have some objective test that will tell us that thyroid function is perfectly normal by a measurement separate from thyroid function tests — for example, a new blood test measuring a chemical that we don't even know about yet, or a nonblood test.

If you have symptoms of hypothyroidism and are taking T4 hormone replacement alone, ask your doctor to prescribe a small dose of T3. You may do better on the combination.

Preventing the Regrowth of Thyroid Cancer

If you have had thyroid cancer, you have probably had thyroid surgery followed by irradiation to eliminate the remaining thyroid tissue. Now you want to prevent any regrowth of thyroid cancer. This is accomplished by taking sufficient thyroid hormone to suppress the production of thyroid-stimulating hormone. This means the goal is for your TSH level to drop below the normal range. The lower level of the normal range is about 0.5, so you want a reading of 0.3 or below to be sure your thyroid isn't being stimulated.

But how low is too low? If a reading of 0.3 is good, would a reading of 0.1 be better? A study published in *Thyroid* in 1999 addressed this issue. The researchers had two groups of cancer patients: One group's TSH levels were suppressed to below 0.1; the other group's TSH levels were kept between 0.4 and 0.1. The study found that residual thyroid tissue was no more suppressed when the TSH was less than 0.1 than when it was less than 0.4. The researchers concluded that thyroid cancer patients should receive suppressive doses of T4 but that greater suppression is no better than lesser degrees of suppression.

The advantage of taking the least suppressive dose of thyroid hormone possible is that you have less risk of developing osteoporosis or rapid heartbeats, particularly if you are middle-aged or older.

Anticipating Drug Interactions

So many drugs interact with thyroid hormones that you must check with your doctor whenever you are placed on a new medication or taken off an old medication (see Chapter 10).

Your thyroid function can be affected not only when you start a new medication, but also if you are taken off an old medication or the dosage is changed significantly.

The way to avoid a problem is to perform (or have your doctor perform) a search for interactions between thyroid hormone and the drugs you'll be taking.

Drugs can affect thyroid function at any level. They can increase or decrease the release of thyrotrophin-releasing hormone, which affects how much thyroid-stimulating hormone (TSH) your body creates. They can increase or decrease the release of thyroid hormone from the thyroid. They can change the ratio of T4 hormone versus T3. They can affect the uptake of thyroid hormone by cells. They can increase or decrease the action of thyroid hormone within the cells.

The major drugs that you should be concerned about are the following, which I discuss in Chapter 10:

- Lithium
- Amiodarone

- ✔ Estrogen
- ✔ Steroids
- ✔ Aspirin (in doses greater than 3,000 milligrams)
- ✔ Iron tablets
- ✔ Iodine
- ✔ Propranolol

Chances are that you will take one or more of these drugs in your lifetime.

Just about every drug affects thyroid function in one way or another. Fortunately, most of the effects can be overcome by your thyroid gland making some adjustment. But if you're on a fixed treatment dose of thyroid hormone, your thyroid cannot adjust as it would normally. It's wise to have your thyroid function tested four to six weeks after you start a new medication or stop an old one.

Protecting Your Thyroid from Radiation

One million or more Americans received neck irradiation for various conditions in the years between 1920 and 1960, and they are at higher risk for thyroid cancer. Close to 10 percent of people who were so treated have developed thyroid cancer to date.

If you received irradiation to your neck area as a child because of enlarged tonsils, acne, an enlarged thymus, or some other condition, you are at increased risk for thyroid cancer and should inform your doctor.

If you have had any kind of radiation treatment to your head, chest, or neck in the past, you should perform the "Neck Check" described earlier in the chapter. If you feel something unusual in shape or size, see your doctor. If you do not, see your doctor anyway because changes may be very subtle and the incidence of thyroid cancer is definitely higher if you have been irradiated. The exception here is that radiation treatment for hyperthyroidism does *not* increase your risk of cancer.

A thyroid scan or a thyroid ultrasound (see Chapter 4) should find any significant abnormality that exists. If one is found, the usual next step is a fine needle biopsy of the thyroid.

What about follow-up if nothing is found? It's probably a good idea to have an examination of your thyroid on at least an annual basis if you have a history of thyroid exposure to radiation.

Even those of us who were never exposed to radiation as part of a medical treatment need to be aware of the risks of radiation. That's because as our sources of fossil fuel for energy are used up, like it or not, we will probably turn more and more to nuclear energy.

You want to be prepared to avoid taking in a lot of radioactive iodine if a nuclear accident occurs at the power plant near you. Fortunately, the Nuclear Regulatory Commission takes this threat seriously. It has arranged to have stockpiles of iodine available to take in the event of a nuclear accident. By taking a large dose of iodine daily for several days, you block the uptake of iodine into the thyroid.

The other thing you can do to protect yourself is to stay indoors. The radiation cannot affect you if you don't come in contact with it.

Exposure of your thyroid to radiation in the past (other than for treatment for hyperthyroidism) definitely increases your risk of thyroid cancer. However, should cancer occur, it's no more dangerous than thyroid cancer not associated with radiation, as long as it's treated properly.

Keeping Up-to-Date with Thyroid Discoveries

This book is an excellent start in your quest for knowledge about the thyroid gland and how it affects you. Most of the information here will be useful for at least 10 years or so. Given the pace of research, however, a book cannot keep you completely up-to-date with new findings about thyroid physiology and pathology. You need to seek them out for yourself. Where do you look?

An obvious start is to wait for an updated version of this book, which will generally have all the important information since the last publication. You can also try the Internet.

In Appendix B, you find the Internet sites that I believe are most accurate and reliable with respect to thyroid function and disease. The Web sites of large organizations like the American Association of Clinical Endocrinologists, the American Thyroid Association, the American Association of Endocrine Surgeons, and the American Association of Thyroid Surgeons are listed.

You also find smaller sites belonging to individuals and groups who have various thyroid conditions or are advocates for those conditions. You can learn a great deal about the experience of having a particular thyroid disease by reading their comments.

There are several government sites that provide a ton of free information about the thyroid. Likewise, there are many institutions of higher learning that want to provide information with the hope that you will seek out their specialists for your ongoing care.

The various drug companies that make thyroid medications have Web sites that contain information especially about their products and often general information about the thyroid as well.

If you speak French, go to the site of the Thyroid Foundation of Canada, where you can find everything you want to know in a French version. This site also has an International Directory of Thyroid-related Organizations. Among the countries listed are Denmark, Germany, Italy, Japan, and the Netherlands.

So many different organizations provide the same information about the thyroid that I often wonder why some of them don't pool their resources to provide one major source. I suppose too many egos are involved to take this logical step, but I still think it's a good idea. Perhaps you are thinking, "Why, Dr. Rubin, with all this information available, did you bother to write this book?" My answer is, of course, that this book is unique. There's no other one quite like it, believe me.

Part VI
Appendixes

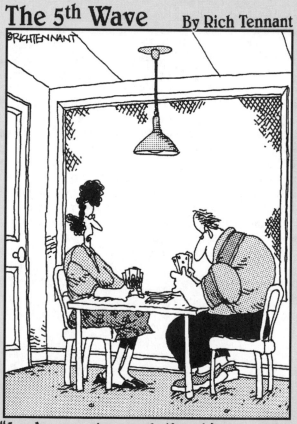

The 5th Wave   By Rich Tennant

"Look- an abnormal thyroid can make you irritable, nervous, and weak in the upper arms. But you can't blame it for the rotten game of gin you're playing."

In this part . . .

Appendix A is a glossary of the terms you encounter as you read and hear about the thyroid gland, its function, and its diseases. All the strange words you meet for the first time in the text of the book are listed here and defined. Appendix B shows you where to look for more information as well as the latest research findings on the thyroid. There is a huge amount of research focusing on every aspect of normal thyroid function and abnormal thyroid conditions. This book gives you a good working knowledge of the subject, but there is always more to know, and these Web sites are where to find it.

Appendix A

A Glossary of Key Terms

Acute thyroiditis: A bacterial infection of the thyroid.

Allele: One of two or more genes that determine which enzyme will be made or which body characteristic will prevail.

Antigen: A foreign protein that prompts the production of antibodies to destroy it.

Autoimmune thyroiditis: Inflammation of the thyroid associated with the production of antibodies against thyroid tissue.

Beta blocking agent: One of a group of drugs given to block some of the adverse effects of excess thyroid hormone.

Chorionic gonadotrophin: A hormone made by the placenta that shares some properties with thyroid-stimulating hormone.

Chromosome: One of 23 pairs in the nucleus of every human cell that carry all the genes that determine the characteristics of the body.

Chronic thyroiditis: Another name for *autoimmune thyroiditis.*

Cretinism: A syndrome affecting children; its most outstanding feature is mental retardation that results from a lack of iodine during pregnancy.

Cyst: A sac-like structure containing fluid.

Cytomel: A brand name for T3 medication.

Dominant gene: The gene that determines which particular enzyme or body characteristic will be expressed when two different genes are present.

Ectopic thyroid: Thyroid tissue found in an abnormal site, such as the base of the tongue.

Exopthalmus: Eye disease associated with Graves' disease.

Fine needle aspiration biopsy (FNAB): The process of putting a tiny needle into tissue, in this case the thyroid, for the purpose of determining the nature of that tissue. This process is particularly helpful for identifying thyroid cancer.

Free thyroxine (FT4): The tiny fraction of the T4 hormone that is not bound to protein and is therefore available to enter cells.

Free thyroxine index (FTI): An obsolete test once used for determining thyroid function. The product of multiplying the total T4 by the T3 resin uptake.

Free triiodothyronine (FT3): The tiny fraction of the T3 hormone that is not bound to protein and is therefore available to enter cells.

Gestational transient thyrotoxicosis: A brief period of hyperthyroidism during pregnancy that results from the large production of human chorionic gonadotrophin (which acts as a thyroid stimulator).

Goiter: An enlarged thyroid gland.

Graves' disease: An autoimmune condition that combines hyperthyroidism, eye disease, and skin disease.

Hashimoto's thyroiditis: Another name for autoimmune or chronic thyroiditis.

Heterozygous: Possessing two different genes for an enzyme or trait.

Homozygous: Possessing two of the same gene for an enzyme or trait.

Hyperthyroidism: A hyperactive state caused by the excessive production or taking of thyroid hormone.

Hypothyroidism: A hypoactive state produced by the diminished production or intake of thyroid hormone.

Isthmus of the thyroid: The thyroid tissue that connects both lobes of the thyroid.

Leptin: A hormone produced by fat cells that signals the brain that the intake of calories is excessive.

Levothroid: A brand name for synthetic thyroxine (T4).

Levoxyl: A brand name for synthetic thyroxine (T4).

Liothyronine: A generic name for T3 medication.

Liotrix: The generic name for the combination of T3 and T4 medication.

Medullary thyroid cancer: A cancer in the thyroid associated with the cells, called *parafollicular* or *C-cells,* that make a hormone called *calcitonin.*

Multinodular goiter: An enlargement of the thyroid associated with many nodules or outgrowths.

Multiple endocrine neoplasia: Hereditary production of tumors in several endocrine glands — one of the tumors may be a medullary thyroid cancer.

Mutation: An unexpected change in the enzyme or body characteristic produced by an alteration in a particular gene.

Myxedema: Another name for hypothyroidism.

Postpartum thyroiditis: Inflammation of the thyroid after a pregnancy that is associated with thyroid autoantibodies and may go through stages of hyperthyroidism, normal thyroid function, and hypothyroidism. It may resolve or end in hypothyroidism. It is often accompanied by depression.

Pyramidal lobe of the thyroid: An accessory lobe rising from the isthmus of the thyroid.

Recessive gene: A gene that will determine an enzyme or body characteristic only when it is present on both chromosomes. (Otherwise the dominant gene prevails.)

Resin T3 uptake: A test of thyroid function (now obsolete) that provides an assessment of the amount of T4 bound to protein compared to the free T4.

Riedel's thyroiditis: A rare form of thyroid inflammation that is often associated with thyroid antibodies. It results in fibrosis of thyroid tissue, and sometimes parathyroid tissue, with tight adherence to the trachea.

Silent thyroiditis: A form of thyroiditis that is identical to postpartum thyroiditis but can be found at any time of life.

Subacute thyroiditis: A viral inflammation of the thyroid. It is associated with pain in the thyroid.

Subclinical hypothyroidism: An elevation of the TSH, with a normal free T4 level and minimal to no symptoms of hypothyroidism.

Synthroid: A brand name for synthetic thyroxine (T4).

Thiocyanate: A chemical found in some foods that may interfere with thyroid function.

Thyroglobulin: Material in the follicle of the thyroid in which thyroid hormones are stored.

Thyroid agenesis: Failure to produce a thyroid gland.

Thyroid autoantibodies: Proteins that react against the thyroid, sometimes to suppress or destroy it and sometimes to stimulate it.

Thyroid dysgenesis: Failure of the thyroid to grow or move into its proper place in the neck, attached to the trachea below the Adam's apple.

Thyroid hypoplasia: Production of a thyroid gland that is inadequate for the needs of the body.

Thyroid scan and uptake: Use of radioactive iodine to outline the thyroid, determine if tissue is actively producing thyroid hormone, and determine the level of activity of the gland.

Thyroid-stimulating hormone (TSH): A hormone from the pituitary gland that stimulates the thyroid to produce more hormone.

Thyroid storm: A very severe form of hyperthyroidism with high fever and severe sickness. It is a medical emergency.

Thyroid ultrasound: Use of sound waves to outline the thyroid and determine if growths are solid or cystic.

Thyrolar: Brand name for combined synthetic T3 and T4 medication.

Thyrotrophin-releasing hormone (TRH): A hormone from the hypothalamus in the brain that stimulates the production and release of thyroid hormone through thyroid-stimulating hormone (TSH).

Thyroxine (T4): The major thyroid hormone.

Thyroxine-binding protein: Several proteins that bind the T3 and T4 hormones, making them unavailable to enter cells.

Total thyroxine: The sum of the thyroxine bound and unbound to thyroid-binding proteins.

Transient congenital hypothyroidism: Temporary hypothyroidism in newborns that often results from prematurity.

Triiodothyronine (T3): The active form of thyroid hormone.

Unithroid: Brand name for synthetic thyroxine (T4).

Vitiligo: Patchy loss of skin pigment sometimes found in autoimmune diseases.

Appendix B

Sources of More Information

T he Web sites described in this appendix offer a vast array of information on thyroid disease, thyroid research, specialists in the field of thyroid health and disease, and companies that make thyroid products. If you can't find what you are looking for here, it probably doesn't exist. Many of the sites point to other links that provide still more information. All these sites can be accessed from my Web page: www.drrubin.com.

You can generally depend upon the information in these sites (although some of them may point you towards other sites where the information is less reliable). But no matter what you read online, *never* make changes in your thyroid care without consulting your physician.

American Association of Clinical Endocrinologists (www.aace.com). This organization was founded in 1992 to serve as the voice of clinical endocrinologists, those actually seeing patients. The site provides practice guidelines, a calendar of important events in endocrinology, and a place both to find an endocrinologist and for endocrinologists to find a position.

American Association of Endocrine Surgeons (www.endocrinesurgeons.org). This organization is dedicated to the advancement of endocrine surgery, and the site is a place to find a thyroid surgeon.

If you live outside the United States, go to the site of the **International Association of Endocrine Surgeons (www.surgery.nbs.ch/iaes)** and select your home area.

American Thyroid Association (www.thyroid.org). This organization was founded in 1923 to promote research in thyroid disease, to spread new knowledge of thyroid disease, and to guide public policy on issues related to thyroid disease. On this important site, you find patient information and guidelines for physicians.

Asia and Oceania Thyroid Association (www.aota.or.kr). This organization was founded to promote thyroid research and education throughout Asia and Oceania.

Endocrine Society (www.endo-society.org). This organization, founded in 1916, is a leading source for research and information on all branches of *endocrinology,* the study of the glands that produce hormones.

European Thyroid Association (www.eurothyroid.com). This organization of European thyroid specialists promotes research and education about thyroid disease.

Jones Medical Industries, Inc. (www.jmedpharma.com/html/patinfo.html). This site provides patient brochures in English and Spanish on thyroid disease.

Latin American Thyroid Society (www.lats.org). This site is dedicated to thyroid research and knowledge in Latin America.

Mayo Clinic Foundation For Medical Information and Research (www.mayoclinic.com/home?id=SPO.0). This site is an excellent source of patient information on major thyroid conditions.

Medline Plus Thyroid Diseases (www.nlm.nih.gov/medlineplus/thyroiddiseases.html). This service of the National Library of Medicine provides information about thyroid disease management and research.

Merck Thyrolink (www.thyrolink.com). This service of Merck Pharmaceutical Company offers patient information in English, German, and French.

National Graves' Disease Foundation (www.ngdf.org). This support group, now more than ten years old, is dedicated exclusively to Graves' patients.

Online Mendelian Inheritance in Man (www.ncbi.nlm.nih.gov/Omim). This site is a huge database of diseases that are inherited by getting a single gene. If you search by "thyroid," you find all the currently known thyroid disorders in this database.

Society of Nuclear Medicine's Guidelines for Patients Receiving Radioiodine Treatment (www.snm.org/nuclear/radioiodine.html). The site provides exactly what the title says.

Synthroid Information Network (www.synthroid.com). This site was founded by Abbott Laboratories, the makers of Synthroid (a form of thyroxine hormone replacement) to provide information concerning their drug.

Thyroid Federation International (www.thyroid-fed.org). This organization was founded in 1995 to deal with the problems of thyroid disease on a global basis. It's mainly involved in helping people start a thyroid patient organization in their country or locale.

Your Thyroid: Gland Central (www.glandcentral.com/home). This educational resource sponsored by the American Medical Women's Association started its journey around the country at Grand Central Station in New York City. It provides information on all aspects of thyroid disease.

Index

• Q •

• R •

• S •

Prevent, Understand, and Manage Your Diabetes with This Ultimate *For Dummies* Guide!

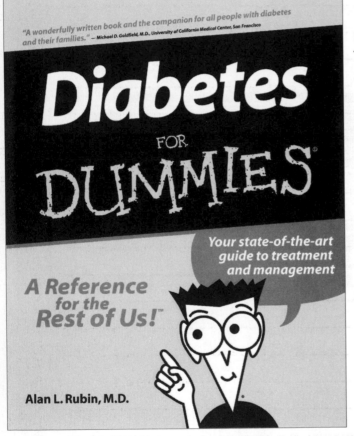

Don't just survive — thrive! That's the message of this state-of-the-art guide to diabetes management.

From causes, symptoms, and side effects to treatment, diet, and exercise, Dr. Alan Rubin helps you understand all types of the disease and delivers sound advice on how to stay fit and feel great.

ISBN: 0-7645-5154-X
$21.99 US • $29.99 CAN • £15.99 UK

<u>**Also Available:**</u>
• Diabetes Cookbook For Dummies
• Allergy & Asthma For Dummies
• Nutrition For Dummies, 2nd Edition

Notes

Notes